W9-CDP-172

Clinical Cases
and OSCEs in
SURGERY

Commissioning Editor: Laurence Hunter
Project Development Manager: Ailsa Laing
Project Manager: Francis Affleck
Designer: Erik Bigland
Illustrations Manager: Bruce Hogarth

Clinical Cases and OSCEs in SURGERY

Manoj Ramachandran

BSc(Hons) MBBS(Hons) MRCS(Eng)
Specialist Registrar in Trauma and Orthopaedics,
North East Thames Rotation, London

Adam Poole

BSc(Hons) MBBS(Hons) MRCS(Eng)
Managing Director, Advanced Medical Courses, London

ELSEVIER
CHURCHILL
LIVINGSTONE

EDINBURGH LONDON NEW YORK OXFORD PHILADELPHIA
ST LOUIS SYDNEY TORONTO 2003

Churchill Livingstone
An imprint of Elsevier Limited

© 2003, Elsevier Limited. All rights reserved.

The right of Manoj Ramachandran and Adam Poole to be identified as authors of
this work has been asserted by them in accordance with the Copyright, Designs
and Patents Act 1988

No part of this publication may be reproduced, stored in a retrieval system, or
transmitted in any form or by any means, electronic, mechanical, photocopying,
recording or otherwise, without either the prior permission of the publishers or a
licence permitting restricted copying in the United Kingdom issued by the
Copyright Licensing Agency, 90 Tottenham Court Road, London W1T 4LP.
Permissions may be sought directly from Elsevier's Health Sciences Rights
Department in Philadelphia, USA: phone: (+1) 215 239 3804, fax: (+1) 215 239
3805, e-mail: healthpermissions@elsevier.com. You may also complete your
request on-line via the Elsevier homepage (http://www.elsevier.com), by
selecting 'Support and contact' and then 'Copyright and Permission'.

First published 2003
    Reprinted 2003, 2004, 2005, 2006, 2007 (twice)

ISBN 978 0 443 07044 0

British Library Cataloguing in Publication Data
A catalogue record for this book is available from the British Library

Library of Congress Cataloguing in Publication Data
A catalogue record for this book is available from the Library of Congress

Note
Medical knowledge is constantly changing. As new information becomes
available, changes in treatment, procedures, equipment and the use of drugs
become necessary. The author, contributor and the publishers have, as far as it is
possible, taken care to ensure that the information given in this text is accurate
and up to date. However, readers are strongly advised to confirm that the
information, especially with regard to drug usage, complies with the latest
legislation and standards of practice.

The Publisher

your source for books,
journals and multimedia
in the health sciences
www.elsevierhealth.com

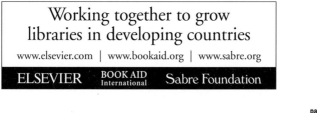

Working together to grow
libraries in developing countries

www.elsevier.com | www.bookaid.org | www.sabre.org

ELSEVIER   BOOK AID International   Sabre Foundation

The
publisher's
policy is to use
**paper manufactured
from sustainable forests**

Printed in China
B/07

This book is designed for candidates sitting both the MRCS clinical section as well as undergraduate clinical examinations in surgery, with the objectives of explaining how the examinations work, and of smoothing the process of passing. The 133 cases in the book are carefully framed to allow interpretation for both short cases and OSCEs. In each case an example of the opening instruction is given, followed by a discussion of the steps required to complete the examination and to pass.

From the start, we set out to create this book from within the context of the examination. The following is a list of the ways in which the ordering, selection of cases, and format of each case are designed to help you to pass.

Structured bays: Cases are listed in clusters that reflect the historical organization of examination cases into areas that examiners have the experience to cover. It is unlikely that a vascular surgeon would feel confident examining an orthopaedic station (particularly at MRCS level).

Common to rare: In OSCEs particularly, commoner cases appear much more frequently than rare cases in the actual clinical exam. This book lists cases in decreasing order of frequency of appearance in the examination within each sub-section; this is denoted by the star rating given to each case, three stars being the most frequently encountered.

Instruction: This is the same for short cases and OSCEs and defines the flow of the case which follows.

Top tips: These are included to emphasize specific areas (often favourites of examiners), which cause confusion or are described differently by different surgeons and teachers.

Finish your examination here: This instruction is added to demonstrate where the marking sheets for an OSCE, or the expectations of a short-case examiner, are likely to conclude. Going beyond this is unlikely to score any further marks and you are more likely to impress by answering some supplemental questions accurately.

Questions and advanced questions: These are designed to fit in with both short-case and OSCE formats, and also cover supplemental questions asked following 'history' scenarios.

Procedures and props: We have included examples of common procedures and props that come up in the skill-based examination format, such as reduction of fractures and description of intramedullary nails and external fixators.

We would be delighted to hear from readers of the book who have an interesting (or unusual) experience in examinations – it helps us to think logically about teaching others on passing the clinical in the future. Please feel free to email us with lists of the cases you were examined on and any specific stories from your examination, and to share your experiences with us. You never know, your experiences may make it into the next edition of the book along with an acknowledgement! The address is **courses@advancedmedicalcourses.com**. Suggestions and feedback will be regularly posted at **www.advancedmedicalcourses.com**.

Thanks for buying and reading this book, and good luck with your exams.

Manoj Ramachandran   London
Adam Poole   2003

ACKNOWLEDGEMENTS

The authors acknowledge the invaluable specialist input given to this text from the following individuals:

Mr Timothy Cheatle MB MCh FRCSI
Consultant Vascular Surgeon, Oldchurch Hospital, Romford, Essex

Dr Paul Dilworth MA DM FRCP
Consultant Respiratory Physician and Honorary Senior Lecturer, Royal Free Hospital, London

Mr Barry Ferris MS FRCS
Consultant Orthopaedic Surgeon, Barnet General Hospital, London

Mr Richard Harrison MS FRCS
Consultant General Surgeon, Barnet General Hospital, London

Mr Charlie Knowles PhD FRCS
Clinical Lecturer and Specialist Registrar in Surgery, Academic Department of Surgery, Royal London Hospital, London

In addition the authors are grateful to the following individuals for their advice:

Rachel Bell, Joanna Broomfield, Gordon Kooiman, Emma Jackson, Will Jackson, Tim McCormick, Ian McDermott, Navin Ramachandran, Sally Richardson, Marc Swan, Hazel Warburton and Dan Weaver

This introduction describes and discusses the different types of assessment of candidates in these examinations and describes the different scenarios that might be presented.

Before going any further – a note of caution. It is often said that the OSCE is completely different from the short case and therefore methods used for preparing for the clinical exam in surgery should be shredded and the process begun from scratch. This is not the case. In fact, there is no fundamental difference between the examination style required – it is only the assessment and marking schemes that are different. Examining an inguinal hernia, or a thyroid lump, or taking a history from a patient with abdominal pain, is the same in each. However, because the OSCE is an 'objective' examination, the marking schedules are much more clearly defined, and deviation (on the part of the examiner) from this is not allowed.

SHORT CASES

Format

At the beginning of the examination, candidates wait in a specific central area to be collected by the examiners, who work in pairs. One asks the questions and the other listens and often makes notes. The examiners lead you round the patients, who are organized in clusters (or 'bays') and choose which patients you meet and in which order.

It is possible to include the description of a prop, or an X-ray or another data-interpretation style question, but these are usually supplemental to the major theme, which is the physical examination of a particular part of a patient. The vast majority of the time will be spent examining the patient and answering questions on the background problem or treatment options.

The examiners choose how many patients you see per bay, which can vary between just one patient to six or seven. The only time limitation is on the whole bay, which may be 10 or 15 minutes. Within that time it is up to the examiner how many patients the candidates see and how deep (and difficult) the supplemental questions become. In Final MB short cases there is usually only one bay, where all the cases are examined, which might be part of a ward or a day surgery unit.

The pros of short cases are that they:

- Allow good candidates to progress rapidly to harder cases or more complex supplemental questions
- Give flexibility for examiners to choose different patients who are waiting in the bay, which is less boring for both examiner and patients
- Allow rapid assessment of clinical skills across areas, e.g. in superficial lesions cases vary from skin lesions to lumps and bumps to thyroid nodules, etc
- Incorporate data interpretation questions, such as chest X-rays, as appropriate
- Test clinical skills across a broad spectrum.

The cons of short cases include that:

- They allow little control of choice of patients an individual examiner picks (except the presence of the co-examiner)
- They can emphasize 'favourite' clinical signs, which may not reflect clinical relevance
- It is difficult to control the marking scheme to ensure transparency and fairness
- They are almost entirely subjective
- It is difficult for candidate to feel confident about doing well (or badly) as the questions tend to get increasingly difficult.

OBJECTIVE STRUCTURED CLINICAL EXAMINATION (OSCE)

Format

The OSCE examination takes the form of a fair, where candidates approach different examiners at different stations (or in different rooms altogether), who test them on specific aspects of the syllabus. The time spent at each station is fixed (often 7–10 minutes) and is the same for every candidate, irrespective of how well, or badly, the candidate is performing at the station. Often a bell rings between stations to let the examiners know to move on to the next candidate. Each OSCE would contain between 10 and 20 stations. The whole examination therefore lasts at least two hours and might be much longer.

In general therefore, an OSCE takes much longer to complete and the time spent on each case (or scenario) is often longer than in the short case format. The marking sheet the examiner has in front of him is pre-set and only allows them to score on specific criteria that are standard for every other examiner as well.

The pros of OSCEs are that:

- The marking scheme is explicit and therefore seen as being 'fairer'
- They reduce inter-examiner variability, and usually mean assessment by a larger number of examiners in total because each scenario is examined by a different clinician
- They allow the possibility of assessment by other doctors (e.g. specialist registrars, medical educators) or other health care professionals
- There tends to be much greater emphasis on patient-centred examining, including communication skills and rapport, i.e. tests greater range of skills (not just clinical examination)
- They allow for much more extensive use of simulated patients – see below.

The cons of OSCEs include that they:

- Are repetitive for examiners and patients – seen as being 'boring' and may lead to error
- Provide little or no scope for examiners to push very strong candidates
- Make it easier to score an average mark, and more difficult to pull out a clear fail or an exceptional candidate
- May present patients as having a certain set of characteristic symptoms or signs, which may not mirror their personal clinical situation
- Usually under-represent unusual cases as they focus on 'common' scenarios.

Simulated patients

Simulated patients are actors. There is a growing industry of simulated patients across medical education. Actors were originally used in teaching and assessment in general practice, and the success of this has led to a huge expansion into other specialties over the last five years. Actors can, of course, be trained and will play a clinical scenario very effectively. Clearly there are drawbacks and their use is confined to history taking and in particular, examination of communication skills. Dummies and mannequins (such as for trauma, breast examination or scrotal examination cases) are also being used much more commonly for the clinical parts of examinations.

The pros of using simulated patients are that they:

- Allow accurate portrayal of 'typical' patients, e.g. response to grief, being given a diagnosis or the treatment of a relative
- Are the most effective way of testing communication skills
- Contribute to discussion of each candidate's performance and even the mark awarded.

The cons of using simulated patients include that:

- They reduce the number of clinical scenarios, and tend to increase history taking and communications stations
- In the same way as practicing basic resuscitation on a dummy, it is different in a real life situation
- It can be difficult to believe if the same actor is used for more than one scenario with the same candidate.

Range of testing

One conclusion about OSCEs is that they don't **just** test clinical examination technique. In fact the areas they test are classified into five different headings:

1 Clinical examinations
2 History taking
3 Data analysis
4 Communication skills technique
5 Practical skills

So how do you know which of these is being tested in a given station?

Clinical examination OSCEs

Who will be at the station (other than examiners)?

- A patient with an identifiable pathology (inguinal hernia, thyroid lump, etc)
- Occasionally a mannequin

What will be available to you?

- Anything required to adequately complete the examination; in a thyroid scenario a glass of water is provided, in a vascular bay a hand-held Doppler probe is provided

How will the scenario begin?

- Normally 'examine...', or 'have a look at...', and you will be directed to the side of the patient's examination couch, or to the area where they are sitting

What kind of questions will be used?

- These will often close in on the pathological problem, especially if the candidate is getting sidetracked with something which is not on the marking sheet for the scenario

What kind of supplemental questions should you expect?

- Supplemental questions might be asked (as included in the chapters of this book) to ascertain background knowledge and understanding of potential treatments.

History taking OSCEs

Who will be at the station (other than examiners)?

- A simulated patient or a real patient

What will be available to you?

- Possibly paper on which to make notes as you take the history

How will the scenario begin?

- You may be asked to gain some information about the symptoms a patient is describing and to formulate a differential diagnosis
- Be aware of the time; you aren't going to be able to complete a whole history but should focus on answering the **exact** question posed, without going into a whole stream of closed questioning

What kind of questions will be used?

- During the scenario none, but if you are interrupted you should take from this that you may be getting side-tracked

What kind of supplemental questions should you expect?

- Again supplemental questions may relate to further parts of the assessment of the patient's symptoms.

Data analysis OSCEs

Who will be at the station (other than examiners)?

- Nobody

What will be available to you?

- Here a 'prop' will be used which might be arterial blood gases, blood laboratory results, joint aspiration results, histopathology results or possibly an X-ray, CT scan or barium series

How will the scenario begin?

- With an explicit instruction to comment on a prop or a set of data

What kind of questions will be used?

- Often very specific (and quite closed) questioning will be used to ensure you understand the clinical significance of any abnormality you pick up

What kind of supplemental questions should you expect?

- Usually these will relate to the clinical situation which has been diagnosed, and are unlikely to relate specifically to history or examination technique.

Communication skills OSCEs

Who will be at the station (other than examiners)?

- Simulated patient

What will be available to you?

- Probably a sheet detailing the communications exercise (which is usually given to you in advance to allow you to prepare)

What kind of questions will be used?

- None, the scenario is a test of your rapport and communication with the patient, not with the examiners

What kind of supplemental questions should you expect?

- None, for the same reason.

Practical skills OSCEs

Who will be at the station (other than the examiners?)

- Nobody

What will be available to you?

- A prop or mannequin

How will the scenario begin?

- With an instruction to demonstrate a specific technique, such as advanced trauma life-support, or suturing, or reduction of a Colles' fracture on the examiner's arm

What kind of questions will be used?

- Usually you talk through as you are proceeding with the case; the only role the examiners have is to ensure that you can adequately perform the specific skill

What kind of supplemental questions should you expect?

- Possibly none.

SCORING SYSTEMS

We set ourselves one objective in writing this book – to help you to pass the examination – and the first stage is to understand under what basis you will be assessed and how you will score marks.

Scoring in short case assessments

As mentioned above this is largely subjective, but marks here are awarded for:

- Introducing yourself to the patient and establishing rapport
- Taking care to appropriately expose the patient (as described in each individual chapter)
- Examining the relevant parts of the body – including starting with the hands
- Accurately identifying the pathological problems (if there are any)
- Coming up with possible further examinations or tests that could be done
- Thinking of a list of differential diagnoses, or a definite diagnosis, and a list of investigations that would tip you towards a particular cause
- Following the train of thought of the examiner, picking up on suggestions and letting yourself be 'taught' technique at the bedside

Scoring in OSCE assessments

This is an objective test, and there is a specific marking sheet, which might look like this:

Bay 1   Superficial lesions
Case 8   Thyroid examination
   Done well = 2, Done adequately = 1, Not done = 0
Elements being assessed:

1 Introdution to patients
2 Adequate exposure
3 Observing neck from front
4 Observing swallow test and protrusion of tongue
5 Palpating neck from behind
6 Checking for cervical lymphadenopathy
7 Percussion and auscultation from the front
8 Mentioning the need to check clinical thyroid status
9 Thanking patient and washing hands

It is possible to come up with a marking scheme for each case in this book by picking out the detail of the examination and making a list of the things you would need to do in order to demonstrate competence. In the same way as in the short cases, there comes a point where you should finish your examination and tell the examiner how you would proceed. This is clearly listed under each case in the book. The examiner indicates if you should continue, and this would imply there are more marks yet to be awarded.

At the end of each case your marks are allotted, then totalled at the end of the entire examination to come up with a score which translates into a pass/fail.

FAILING THE CLINICAL EXAMINATION

Failing a clinical exam is most likely if you are not seen to show due concern for the patient, such as not introducing yourself, not exposing adequately, and not asking permission before examining. The examiners may be trying very hard to give a hint that you are heading in completely the wrong direction. Ignoring these hints, and not listening carefully enough to the question, may also lead to a failed case. Gross lack of knowledge or understanding is the third possibility.

A common mistake in OSCEs is to assume that you pass if you show concern for the patient and establish rapport, making them 'like you'. It isn't as simple as this and at all levels you are also expected to ask questions or examine intelligently and come up with the right answers to most of the questions. You don't fail the whole examination for failing one OSCE though, and one of the most important things to do is brush yourself down after each station and get on with trying to pass the next. We all naturally emphasize the things that haven't gone so well in our minds, and this will tend to psychologically knock you down during OSCEs. Work on ways of concentrating on what you have done well at each station and move on to the next, keeping your mind as fresh and alert as possible.

In the OSCE, reducing as many variables as possible from the assessment reduces the chance that a candidate who should have passed will actually fail (i.e. the false-negative rate). Variables that are reduced (or eliminated) in this format include the following:

- **Intra-examiner variability** – where an examiner (by chance) chooses a 'harder' set of cases for a given candidate compared with the one he examines immediately before or afterwards
- **Inter-examiner variability** – where different examiners have wildly different expectations of the appropriate amount of knowledge required to pass
- **Testing one single modality** – where, instead of just being tested on clinical examination, a range of skills (as above) is examined.

Studies have also been attempted to prove that a 'pass' mark for the OSCE can be more fairly ascertained than in the short cases[1]. Five different medical schools testing students using the same examination were able to prove that by averaging the scores of borderline candidates at each station a passing score for that station could be accurately replicated. There was good agreement between examiners, stations and schools as to the reliable setting of these scores.

WORLDWIDE OSCE?

A recent survey of US surgical educators found that the OSCE is gaining in popularity in US examinations, and produced a list of common cases/scenarios (Table) as used in US OSCE examinations[2]:

Table   Common cases as used in US examinations

Rank	History taking	Physical examination	Data interpretation	Surgical technique
1	Abdominal pain	Acute abdomen	Chest X-Ray	Central line
2	Breast mass	Trauma survey	Abdominal (barium) series	Basic suture skills
3	Gastrointestinal bleeding	Breast examination	CT scan	Bowel anastamosis
4	Bowel obstruction	Peripheral vascular examination	Mammogram	Informed consent

The interest comes not just for UK doctors who are considering studying or working in the US, but is also informative because the process of structuring the OSCE in the USA is largely similar to that the UK. The topics are split into broad headings ('history taking', 'data interpretation', etc) and then individual cases put into the most relevant category. In other educational systems (and the US system is in many ways completely different from the training and educational system in the UK, Australia, New Zealand and most of the rest of the English-speaking countries), a similar process has been followed.

REFERENCES

1 Wilkinson TJ, Newble DI, Frampton CM 2001 Standard setting in an objective structured clinical examination: use of global ratings of borderline performance to determine the passing score. *Medical Education* **35**(11): 1043–1049

2 Cerilli, GJ, Merrick H, Staren ED 2001 Surgical educator preferences regarding key objective structured clinical examination topics. *Journal of Surgical Research* **101**(2): 124–129

CONTENTS

SECTION 1
SUPERFICIAL LESIONS 1

SECTION 2
ABDOMEN AND TRUNK   97

SUPERFICIAL LESIONS

CASE 1   LUMPS AND ULCERS – EXAMINATION   ★ ★ ★

INSTRUCTION

'Examine this lump.'

APPROACH

Every clinical examination in surgery includes the description of a lump. Also, more often than in any other case, the examiners may expect an on-the-spot diagnosis. The description given here of the examination technique is complete and exhaustive, but be prepared to give a diagnosis and to describe the specific features which have led you to this conclusion.

VITAL POINTS

Inspect

- Site – most accurately measured with respect to a fixed landmark such as a bony prominence
- Size – measure the dimension in centimetres

If the lump is large enough, be seen to use a measuring tape/ruler, but do not use a tape on a small lump as it appears awkward.

- Shape
- Skin changes
- Symmetry
- Scars
- Colour

Ask the patient if the lump is tender before proceeding with the examination.

Palpate

- Surface – smooth/irregular
- Edge – well/poorly defined
- Consistency – soft/firm/hard
- Temperature – using the dorsal surface of the examining fingers or hand
- Tenderness
- Transilluminability – using a pen torch on one side of the lump and looking through an opaque tube such as an empty Smarties tube (this is difficult and cumbersome to perform in a well-lit room and we therefore recommend not taking an empty Smarties tube into the exam, especially if the lump is a hydrocele!)
- Pulsatility – place a finger on opposite sides of the lump
  - expansile pulsation = fingers pushed apart
  - transmitted pulsation = fingers pushed in the same direction (usually upwards)

- Compressibility/reducibility – press firmly on the lump and release
  - compressible = lump disappears on pressure but reappears on release, e.g. arteriovenous malformations
  - reducible = lump disappears on pressure but reappears only when another opposite force is applied such as coughing in hernia examination
- Fluctuation (for small lumps) – rest two fingers of one hand on opposite sides of the lump and press the middle of the lump with the index finger of your other hand – if the fingers are moved apart, the lump is fluctuant (*Repeat the test at right angles to the first in order to confirm your findings*). This is also known as Paget's sign (*see* Case 107)
- Fluid thrill – for large lumps – ask the patient to place the edge of his hand on the centre of the lump and then flick one side of it, feeling the other side for a percussion wave (most commonly performed in ascites, Case 57)
- Fixation – decide which plane the lump is in by determining which structures it is attached to, e.g.:
  - skin – see if you can move the skin over the lump
  - muscle – move the lump in two planes perpendicular to each other, ask the patient to then tense the relevant muscle and reassess the motion in the two planes.

Percuss

- Dull/resonant (the latter indicating an air-filled lump)

Auscultate

- Bruits or bowel sounds may be heard

Finish your examination here

Completion

Say that you would like to:

- Examine the draining lymph nodes
- Assess the neurovascular status of the area/limb
- Look for similar lumps elsewhere
- Perform a general examination (as necessary)

TOP TIP

When assessing consistency, imagine:

- Soft to be comparable to the consistency of the flesh of your nostrils (i.e. the ala)
- Firm to that of your nasal septum
- Hard to that of the bridge of your nose

Mnemonic

We use the following mnemonic to remind us what to do with a lump – it is very useful as an aide-memoire for completeness, but does not provide you with the correct order of examination:

Should The Children Ever Find Lumps Readily

S – Size/Site/Shape/Surface/Skin changes/Symmetry/Scars
T – Temperature/Tenderness/Transilluminability
C – Colour/Consistency/Compressibility
E – Edge/Expansility and Pulsatility
F – Fluctuation/Fluid thrill/Fixation
L – Lymph nodes/Lumps elsewhere
R – Resonance/Relations to surrounding structures & their state, e.g. neuro-vascular status

---

A NOTE ON ULCERS
Ulcers should be examined in a similar way to a lump, but important additional points to look for on examination can be remembered in the form of the mnemonic **BEDD**:

B – base. Look for the presence of granulation tissue, slough (i.e. dead tissue) or evidence of malignant change
E – edge. Five types of edges to be aware of are:
  • Sloping = a healing ulcer (usually venous or traumatic)
  • Punched-out = ischaemic or neuropathic (rarely syphilis)
  • Undermined = pressure necrosis or tuberculosis
  • Rolled = basal cell carcinoma
  • Everted = squamous cell carcinoma

D – describe which structure is visualized at the base of the ulcer, e.g. is the ulcer down to fascia, muscle or bone?
D – discharge. Is the discharge serous (clear), sanguinous (blood-stained), serosanguinous (mixed) or purulent (infected)?

Individual ulcers, e.g. arterial, venous, neuropathic, are considered in the appropriate sections.

*** **LIPOMA** **CASE 2**

INSTRUCTION

No specific instruction.

APPROACH

Examine as for any lump (*see* Case 1).

VITAL POINTS

Lipomas can occur anywhere in the body where there are fat cells, although they most commonly occur in the subcutaneous layer of the skin, particularly in the neck and trunk.

Inspect

- Discoid or hemispherical swelling
- May appear lobulated
- Look carefully for scars (may be a recurrent lipoma)

Palpate

- Lobulated surface
- May be soft or firm depending on the nature of the fat within the lipoma and the temperature at which it liquefies
- If soft and large in size, may show fluctuation
- 'Slip sign' – describes the manner in which a lipoma tends to slip away from the examining finger on gentle pressure
- Skin freely mobile over the lipoma (compared with a sebaceous cyst)
- Try and elicit which layer the lipoma is in, e.g. whether subcutaneous or intramuscular (in the latter case, the lipoma disappears on contraction of the relevant muscle)

Completion

Say that you would like to ask the patient:

- How the lipoma affects their lives, e.g. cosmetic symptoms
- Whether they have noticed similar lumps elsewhere

QUESTIONS

(a) What is a lipoma?

A lipoma is a benign tumour consisting of mature fat cells. Multiple, painful lipomas are known as adiposis dolorosa or Dercum's disease, and are associated with peripheral neuropathy.

(b) Do lipomas undergo malignant change?

- It is thought that malignant change in a lipoma does not occur
- Liposarcomas arise de novo and usually occur in an older age-group in deeper tissues of the lower limbs

(c) How would you treat a lipoma?

- Non-surgical – reassure and 'watch and wait'
- Surgical – if the patient wants it removed, e.g. pain, cosmesis. Some surgeons remove lipomas using suction lipolysis via a small, remote incision. Usually this is performed under local anaesthetic. However, 'nuchal' lipomas have extremely fibrous septae and are difficult to excise, and any lipoma close to a joint may communicate with the joint and it may not be possible to excise it under local anaesthetic.

ADVANCED QUESTIONS

(a) Do you know of any variants of lipomas or syndromes associated with lipomas?

- Angiolipomas, which have a prominent vascular component
- Hibernomas, which consist of brown fat cells similar to those seen in hibernating animals
- Cowden's disease – association of lipomas, palmoplantar keratoses, multiple facial papules, oral papillomatoses and vitiligo, with involvement of the thyroid and digestive tract
- Bannayan–Zonana syndrome – rare autosomal dominant hamartomatous disorder, characterized by multiple lipomas, macrocephaly and haemangiomas

(b) How are liposarcomas classified?

- Liposarcomas can be classified pathologically into three main groups:
  1. well-differentiated liposarcoma, characterized by ring or long markers, chromosomes derived from the long arm of chromosome 12
  2. myxoid and round cell (poorly differentiated myxoid) liposarcoma, characterized in most cases by a reciprocal translocation t(12;16)(q13;p11)
  3. pleomorphic liposarcoma, characterized by complex karyotypes

> *F. X. Dercum (1856–1931)*. North American neurologist, born in Philadelphia

FURTHER READING

Dei Tos A P (2000) Liposarcoma: new entities and evolving concepts. *Ann Diagn Pathol* **4**(4): 252–66.

Chen D Y, Wang C M, Chan H L (1998) Hibernoma. Case report and literature review. *Dermatol Surg* **24**(3): 393–5.

http://www.lipoman.com – the website of Dr Steven J Kalamara MD, an expert on suction lipolysis and the man affectionately nicknamed 'Lipoman'!

*** **SEBACEOUS CYST** **CASE 3**

INSTRUCTION

No specific instruction.

APPROACH

Examine as for any lump (*see* Case 1).

VITAL POINTS

Inspect

- Smooth hemispherical swelling
- Usually solitary
- Found most commonly on the face, trunk, neck and scalp
- Punctum present at apex of cyst in 50%

Palpate

- Smooth surface
- Firm to soft on palpation
- Punctum may exhibit plastic deformation on palpation
- All sebaceous cysts are attached to the skin, therefore the cyst does not move independently from the skin

Completion

Say that you would like to ask the patient:

- How the cyst affects their lives, e.g. cosmetic symptoms
- Whether they have noticed similar lumps elsewhere

QUESTIONS

(a) What are the complications of a sebaceous cyst?

- Infection – frequent complication, there may be an associated discharge
- Ulceration
- Calcification (trichilemmal cysts (see below) – this may cause the cyst to feel hard on palpation)
- Sebaceous horn formation (hardening of a slow discharge of sebum for a wide punctum)
- Malignant change

(b) How would you treat a sebaceous cyst?

- Non-surgical – may be left alone if small and asymptomatic
- Surgical – to prevent recurrence, complete excision of cyst and its contents is required which requires removal of an elliptical portion of skin containing the punctum

ADVANCED QUESTIONS

(a) What are the different histological subtypes of sebaceous cysts?

Two types of cysts are recognised according to their histological features:
- Epidermal cyst (EC) – thought to arise from the infundibular portions of hair follicles
- Trichilemmal cysts (TC) – thought to arise from hair follicle epithelium and so are most common on the scalp, and are frequently multiple; these cysts have an autosomal dominant mode of inheritance

(b) What is a Cock's peculiar tumour?

Proliferating trichilemmal cysts are usually solitary, occur on the scalp in 90% of cases, and can grow to a large size and ulcerate. Clinically and histologically, they may resemble a squamous cell carcinoma, in which case it is known as a Cock's peculiar tumour. Very rarely, malignant transformation can occur

(c) What is Gardner's syndrome?

Multiple epidermal cysts may be part of Gardner's syndrome, which is also associated with:
- Adenomatous polyposis of the large bowel
- Multiple osteomata of the skull
- Desmoid tumours

Note that Gardner's syndrome is now part of the spectrum of familial polyposis coli syndromes, which includes familial adenomatous polyposis

---

E. Cock (1805–1892), English surgeon at Guy's Hospital, who was the nephew of Sir Astley Cooper.
E. J. Gardner (born 1909), American geneticist and Professor of Zoology, Utah State University.

FURTHER READING

Dastgeer G M (1991) Sebaceous cyst excision with minimal surgery. *Am Fam Physician* **43**(6): 1956–60.

http://www.theberries.ns.ca/Archives/Sebaceous_Cyst.html – how to surgically excise a sebaceous cyst.
http://www.intelihealth.com/IH/ihtIH/WSIHW000/9339/9779.html – information for patients on sebaceous cysts.

INSTRUCTION

'Examine this gentleman's hand.'

APPROACH

Expose to elbows and ask the patient to place his hands palm upwards on a pillow (if available).

VITAL POINTS

Ganglia can occur anywhere in the body, although they are commonly found around the wrist, on the dorsum of the hand and on the dorsum of the ankle. In fact, the most common soft-tissue mass found in the hand is a ganglion.

Inspect

- Usually single
- Hemispherical swelling
- Look carefully for scars (may be recurrent)

Palpate

- Smooth surface
- May be multiloculated
- May be soft and fluctuant (especially if large) or firm (if small with tense, viscous contents)
- Associated with a synovial lined structure such as a tendon or joint
- Weakly transilluminable due to its viscous fluid contents

Completion

Say that you would like to ask the patient:

- How the ganglion affects their lives, e.g. cosmetic symptoms
- Whether they have noticed similar lumps elsewhere
- Which hand is dominant (considering treatment options)
- Their occupation (also to consider treatment options)

QUESTIONS

(a) What is a ganglion?

A ganglion is a cystic swelling related to a synovial lined cavity, either a joint or a tendon sheath. The origin of ganglia is controversial – they are seen as a pocket of synovium communicating with the joint or tendon sheath, or as a myxomatous degeneration of fibrous tissue.

(b) What is the differential diagnosis?

- Bursae
- Cystic protrusions from synovial cavity of arthritic joints
- Benign giant cell tumours of the flexor sheath (indistinguishable from flexor sheath ganglia)
- Rarely, malignant swellings, e.g. synovial sarcoma

(c) How would you treat a ganglion?

- Non-surgical – 'watch and wait', or aspiration followed by 3 weeks of immobilization (successful in 30–50% of patients). The old method of striking the ganglion with the family Bible is now out of favour!
- Surgical – complete excision to include the neck of the ganglion at its site of origin

(d) What complications are associated with surgical treatment of a ganglion?

- Wound complications, e.g. scar, haematoma, infection
- Recurrence – can be as high as 20% but as low as 5% if care is taken to completely excise the neck
- Damage to adjacent neurovascular structures

FURTHER READING

Thornburg L E (1999) Ganglions of the hand and wrist. *J Am Acad Orthop Surg* 7(4): 231–8.

http://www.med.und.nodak.edu/users/jwhiting/ganglia.html – information for patients.

*** LUMPS AND ULCERS – HISTORY | CASE 5

INSTRUCTION

'Ask this gentleman a few questions about his lump/ulcer.'

APPROACH

It is extremely common in short cases at Finals, OSCE examinations, and at the MRCS to be asked to take a focused history from a patient presenting with relatively common problems. Listen carefully to the instruction. After introducing yourself and establishing the patient's name and age, go straight to questions about the lump or ulcer. When you have done this, you may continue on to further relevant surgical questions such as fitness for anaesthesia. The examiner will usually stop you once you have extracted the necessary information. You may not always be asked to continue to examine the patient – so it is a mistake to make any assumption about this.

> TOP TIP 1
> If the examiner tells you the patient's name, then do not embarrass yourself by asking his name again – this only shows that you have not been listening to the examiner!

VITAL POINTS

You should ask the following questions about the lump/ulcer:

Onset

- When did you first notice the lump?
- What made you notice it?
- Were there any predisposing events? (e.g. trauma, insect bite)

Continued symptoms

- How does it bother you? (i.e. what symptoms does it cause?) – ask particularly about pain
- Has it changed since you first noticed it? (e.g. colour, shape and size changes are important in malignant melanoma)
- Have you noticed any other lumps?
- Has it ever disappeared or healed?

Treatments and cause

- What treatments have you had in the past for this lump?
- What do you think is the cause of the lump?

You will usually find that as you extract the relevant information, the examiner will move you onto the examination relatively quickly.

> TOP TIP 2
> When asked to take a history, keep eye contact with the patient throughout your questioning. Don't stare at the lump – the examiner will probably notice!

CASE 6   NECK EXAMINATION – GENERAL   ***
                               APPROACH

INSTRUCTION

'Examine this gentleman's neck.'

APPROACH TO THE NECK

- Note that the patient is usually sitting in a chair and may have a glass of water next to him
- If there is a glass of water, be prepared to examine the thyroid gland in full
- Expose the whole neck down to both clavicles – this may necessitate undoing the top buttons of a shirt or even taking off a polo neck jumper
- Ask the patient to remove any jewellery present

> TOP TIP
> The examiners may try to catch you out by placing the patient on a chair with its back against the wall. Your first move is to ask the patient to stand up and move the chair away from the wall, allowing you to access and examine the patient's neck from behind.

VITAL POINTS

Inspect (FROM THE FRONT)

- Site of the lump, e.g. midline, supraclavicular fossa
- Other features on inspection of the lump, e.g. size, skin changes, scars (*see* Case 1)

Protrusion of the tongue

- Ask the patient to open his mouth and stick his tongue out as far as possible
- If the lump moves on protrusion of the tongue, it is likely to be a thyroglossal cyst (this is because the cyst is usually related to the base of the tongue by a patent or fibrous track which runs through the central portion of the hyoid bone) – proceed with examination of a thyroglossal cyst (*see* Case 31)
- A thyroid lump does not move on protrusion of the tongue

Swallowing

- Place the glass of water in the patient's hands
- Ask him to take a sip of water, hold it in his mouth and swallow when you ask him to
- As he swallows, inspect the lump – if it moves on swallowing, it is likely to originate from the thyroid gland
- Note that thyroglossal cysts also move on swallowing, so ask the patient to stick his tongue out before proceeding with the thyroid gland examination (*see* Case 8)

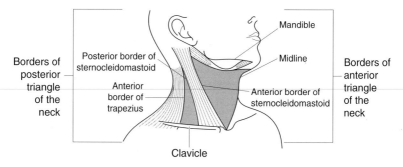

Fig. 1 Posterior and anterior triangles of the neck.

Palpate (FROM THE BACK)

- The neck is best (and first) palpated from behind the patient
- Be as gentle as possible as you are unable to watch the patient's face for pain
- Use the fingertips of both hands to elicit the physical signs
- Begin by showing the examiner that you know the borders of the two main triangles of the neck and tell him which triangle the lump is in (Fig. 1)

The *anterior triangle* of the neck is bordered by the anterior border of sternocleidomastoid, the midline and the ramus of the mandible.

The *posterior triangle* of the neck is bordered by the anterior border of trapezius, the clavicle and the posterior border of sternocleidomastoid.

- Next, determine whether the lump is solid or cystic. You should now be ready to consider the differential diagnosis (Table 1)

Table 1   Differential diagnosis of neck lumps

Position	Solid	Cystic
Midline	Thyroid swelling (Case 8)	Thyroglossal cyst (Case 31)
Anterior triangle	Lymphadenopathy (Case 7)	Branchial cyst (Case 29)
	Chemodectoma (Case 38)	Cold abscess (secondary to tuberculosis)
Posterior triangle	Lymphadenopathy	Pharyngeal pouch (Case 36) Cystic hygroma (Case 37)
Within sternocleidomastoid	Sternocleidomastoid tumour (see below)	

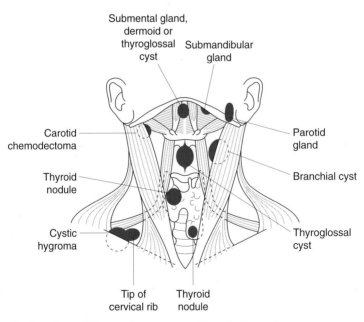

Fig. 2   Locations of the most common swellings in the neck.

Continuing the examination

If at this stage you think that the lump is thyroid in origin you should proceed to examine the thyroid gland in full (*see* Case 8).

If you have attempted a differential diagnosis you should be prepared to offer additional 'evidence' for your suggestions – see individual cases.

If you have not found a lump at this stage you should examine the neck thoroughly using the up and down technique as in Table 2.

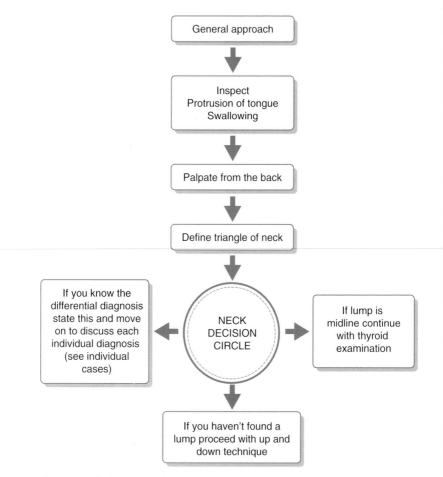

Fig. 3 'Neck decision circle' approach to examination of the neck.

Table 2   The up and down technique

Stage 1	Palpate from the chin backwards to below the ears
Stage 2	Move your hands behind the ears and palpate DOWN the anterior border of sternocleidomastoid to the clavicle
Stage 3	Move laterally along the clavicle and then UP the posterior border of sternocleidomastoid
Stage 4	Finish by palpating the back of the scalp for occipital nodes

Examination of cervical lymph nodes

The cervical lymph nodes (Fig. 4) are best examined using the 'up-and-down' technique:

- Use gentle rotating movements of the fingertips – this allows you to palpate even the smallest nodes
- If the patient tries to help you by raising their chin, ask him to drop his chin – this makes the examination easier by relaxing the anterior neck muscles

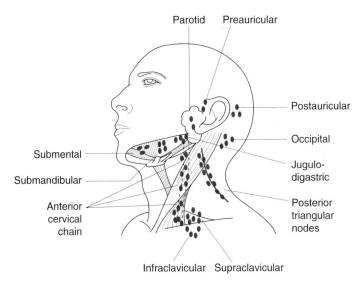

Fig. 4   Typical grouping of lymph nodes.

- Begin by moving from the chin backwards, palpating the submental, submandibular and parotid glands and pre-auricular nodes
- Move your fingers behind the ears and feel the mastoid (post-auricular) nodes
- Go down the anterior border of the sternocleidomastoids, feeling the anterior triangular nodes, including the jugulodigastric (tonsillar) node
- Move laterally along the clavicular region, feeling for both supraclavicular and infraclavicular nodes
- Move up the posterior border of the sternocleidomastoids, feeling the posterior triangular nodes
- Finish by palpating the occipital nodes at the back of the neck

Palpate (from the front)

- Confirm your findings if necessary by feeling the lump from the front, watching the patient's face carefully for signs of discomfort

Percussion and auscultation

See individual cases

Finish your examination here

Footnote

Sternomastoid tumour – an ischaemic contracture of a segment of the muscle seen to appear in the first 1–2 weeks after birth (following a complicated or breech birth) and normally disappearing over the first 4–6 months of life. Babies may present with a torticollis. With early diagnosis, non-surgical treatment with active stimulation and passive stretching and occasionally using *Botulinum toxin* injections; with late diagnosis, may require surgery.

*** CERVICAL LYMPHADENOPATHY CASE 7

INSTRUCTION

'Examine this gentleman's neck.'

APPROACH

Approach as you would a neck examination (*see* Case 6). Note that cervical lymph nodes are the commonest neck lumps found in the clinical cases.

Inspection, protrusion of the tongue, swallowing, palpation

(*See* Case 6)

Additional points on inspection

- Site of the lump, e.g. midline, supraclavicular fossa
- Other features on inspection of any lump, e.g. size, skin changes, scars (*see* Case 1)

Additional points on palpation (FROM THE BACK)

- Use the 'up-and-down' routine as detailed in Case 6 to examine thoroughly for cervical lymphadenopathy
- Remember also that the lymph nodes should be examined as for any other lump (*see* Case 1) and particularly note
  - consistency – tends to be firm but may be rubbery
  - number – solitary, multiple or matted to each other
  - fixation – skin tethering in tuberculous nodes or malignancy

Finish your examination here

Completion

Say that you would like to:

- Examine the face and scalp carefully for a primary site of infection or neoplasia
- Perform a full examination of the ear, nose and throat (say that you would request a formal full ENT examination) and the thyroid gland
- Examine the rest of the lymphoreticular system, including palpation of the abdomen for hepatomegaly and splenomegaly
- Look for a primary site of infection or neoplasia above the umbilicus, e.g. chest examination
- In a female patient a breast examination would also be indicated as breast malignancy can metastasize to the neck

QUESTIONS

(a) What questions would you like to ask this gentleman?

Concentrate on:

- Symptoms from the lump itself, for example the duration, pain (e.g. in lymphomas pain is experienced on alcohol ingestion, although this is not specific to lymphomas), other lumps elsewhere
- General symptoms, e.g. night sweats, loss of appetite, loss of weight
- Local symptoms, e.g. intraoral diseases such as tooth decay
- Systemic disease, e.g. serious medical illnesses, previous surgical operations (thinking of neoplasia)
- Social history – ethnic origin (patients from high-risk areas for TB including the Indian subcontinent), foreign travel, contact with animals (cat scratch fever), risk-factors for HIV infection

(b) What causes of cervical lymphadenopathy do you know of?

Think of the mnemonic LIST when considering this answer:

L Lymphoma and leukaemia
I Infection (see below)
S Sarcoidosis
T Tumours (primary/secondary)

Infectious causes can, as always, be further subclassified:

- Bacterial
  - tonsillitis, dental abscess (β-haemolytic streptococcus)
  - tuberculosis
- Viral
  - cytomegalovirus
  - infectious mononucleosis (Epstein-Barr virus)
  - Human Immunodeficiency Virus
- Protozoal
  - toxoplasmosis

(c) How would you investigate this gentleman?

- Blood tests:
  - haematological – full blood count, erythrocyte sedimentation rate
  - biochemical – thyroid function tests, angiotensin converting enzyme levels which may be raised in sarcoidosis
  - serological – 'monospot' or Paul–Bunnell test looking for atypical mononuclear cells in infectious mononucleosis
- Radiological:
  - ultrasound
  - CT scan
  - MRI scan
- Fine-needle aspiration cytology (FNAC):
  - false-positive rate 0–3%, false-negative rate 1–10%
  - errors reduced by experience of clinician and cytologist

ADVANCED QUESTIONS

(a) What results might you expect from the FNAC and how would you proceed?

- If malignant:
  - is it squamous cell carcinoma? – Do not perform open lymph node excision biopsy (spoils the field for subsequent block dissection of the neck and may reduce survival), refer to ENT surgeon for full assessment to include panendoscopy to find a primary tumour. Random biopsies from multiple sites may be needed, along with sputum cytology and chest X-ray
  - is it adenocarcinoma? Continue to open lymph node excision biopsy and look for primary from breast or intra-abdominal viscera such as pancreas or stomach
  - is it lymphoma? Continue to open lymph node excision biopsy as a whole node is required for detailed histology and marker studies

- If inflammatory:
  - is it tuberculosis? Do not perform open lymph node excision biopsy (may result in chronic sinus formation) – treat as for tuberculosis
  - is it another infectious or inflammatory disorder? Continue to open lymph node excision biopsy and treat according to underlying cause

(b) What surgical options are available in the management of cervical lymphadenopathy?

- Open lymph node excision biopsy:
  - best performed under general anaesthesia
  - beware biopsy in the posterior triangle due to risk of damaging the spinal accessory nerve which is quite superficial – damage leads to shoulder and arm pain, paralysis of trapezius and winging of the scapula
  - in addition patients should be warned of damage to the facial nerve if the surgical approach includes dissection around the parotid gland
- Block dissection of the neck:
  - classic operation involves removing the sternomastoid, jugular vein and accessory nerve
  - limited dissection is now in favour (supra-omohyoid only in oral and oropharyngeal carcinoma and lateral only in hypopharyngeal and pharyngeal tumours) in conjunction with radiotherapy
- Radical neck dissection:
  - clear all lymphatic tissue from mandible above to clavicle below, and from the midline to the anterior border of the trapezius laterally
  - incisions used include the 'wineglass', the standard Y and the McFee incision
  - details of the dissection itself are beyond postgraduate level

---

J. R. Paul (1893–1971). North American physician and pathologist.
W. W. Bunnell (1902–1966). North American physician.
Thomas Hodgkin (1798–1866). English physician, St. Thomas's Hospital and Curator of the Pathology Museum at Guy's Hospital.
M. A. Epstein (1921–). English physician and Professor of Pathology, Bristol
Yvonne Barr (1932–). English physician.

FURTHER READING

Peters T R, Edwards K M (2000) Cervical lymphadenopathy and adenitis. *Pediatr Rev* **21**(12): 399–405.

*** **THYROID EXAMINATION**   **CASE 8**

INSTRUCTION

'Examine this lady's thyroid gland.'

APPROACH

- See general approach to examination of the neck (Case 6)
- As you start the examination, you should be looking for clues of thyroid dysfunction such as:
  - a hoarse voice (recurrent laryngeal nerve palsy)
  - warm and sweaty hands (hyperthyroidism)

TOP TIP
Divide the examination of the thyroid gland into three parts:
- The thyroid itself
- Structures around the thyroid gland:
  - trachea and oesophagus
  - recurrent laryngeal nerve
  - cervical lymph nodes
- The thyroid status

PART 1: THE THYROID ITSELF

Inspection, protrusion of the tongue, swallowing, palpation

See Case 6.

Additional points on inspection

- Obvious midline lump (see footnote for definition of goitre)
- Scars – horizontal skin crease incision is most common following previous thyroid surgery
- Raised jugular venous pulse – due to neck vein obstruction from mass effect

Additional points on palpation (FROM THE BACK)

- Ask the patient to stick her tongue out again – checking for a thyroglossal cyst – while gently palpating the thyroid gland
- Repeat the swallow test, asking her to take another sip of water, hold it in her mouth and swallow when you ask her to. Feel the thyroid gland rise, proving the mass arises from the thyroid.
- Describe the features of the lump – gently push on one edge of the lump so that you can palpate the other edge with ease (*be gentle!*) – feel particularly for:
  - size
  - tenderness

 – mobility
 – consistency
- Most importantly, try to work out whether the thyroid is:
  – diffusely enlarged or
  – nodular

TOP TIP – A SCHEME FOR THYROID ENLARGEMENT

Diffuse enlargement

- Toxic (i.e. hyperthyroid) = Grave's disease (*see* Case 11)
- Non-toxic (i.e. euthyroid) = Simple colloid goitre (*see* Case 11), thyroiditis, e.g. Hashimoto's, de Quervain's or Reidel's; in these cases the thyroid may be tender

Nodular enlargement

- Solitary nodule (*see* Case 9)
- Multinodular goitre (*see* Case 10)
- Move on to examining the cervical lymph nodes performing the 'up-and-down' routine (*see* Case 6)

Palpate (FROM THE FRONT)

- Confirm your findings if necessary by feeling the lump from the front, watching the patient's face carefully for signs of discomfort

PART 2: STRUCTURES AROUND THE THYROID

- Gently palpate the trachea for deviation (from a large goitre – see below) and ask the patient if she has had any problems swallowing or noticed any change in her voice – this completes the examination of the structures around the thyroid gland
- Percuss over the sternum from the notch downwards listening for a change in percussion note if there is retrosternal extension – this is very rare
- You could ask the patient to repeat a sentence that you read out in order to listen for the hoarse voice characteristic of a previously damaged or infiltrated recurrent laryngeal nerve

PART 3: THYROID STATUS

This includes examination of the hands and eyes, and occasionally knowing other areas to examine for more evidence of thyroid dysfunction. You will not usually be asked to continue to perform this part of the examination if the patient has normal thyroid status (is euthyroid)

Move on to the hands

There are seven signs to look for in the hands:

- Increased sweating (due to hyperthyroidism)
- Palmar erythema (due to hyperthyroidism)
- Thyroid acropachy (a feature of Grave's disease – *see* Case 11) – also known as pseudoclubbing
- Onycholysis (Plummer's nails – *see* Case 10)
- Areas of vitiligo (white patches of skin +/– hyperpigmented borders, seen in association with autoimmune disorders such as Grave's disease)
- Pulse – tachycardia or atrial fibrillation in hyperthyroidism, bradycardia in hypothyroidism
- Fine tremor – best demonstrated by placing a sheet of paper on the outstretched hands with palms facing downwards

Proceed to the eyes

There are also seven signs to look for in the eyes, the latter six being associated with Grave's disease (*see* Case 11):

- Loss of hair on outer third of eyebrows (hypothyroidism)
- Lid retraction – raised upper eyelid but the whiteness of the sclera is not visible around the iris – also known as Dalrymple's sign

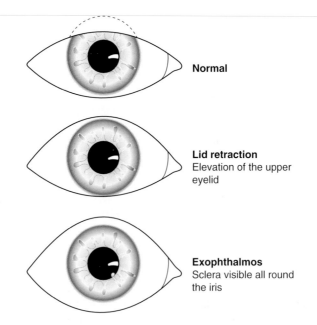

Normal

Lid retraction
Elevation of the upper eyelid

Exophthalmos
Sclera visible all round the iris

Fig. 5 Eye signs in Grave's disease.

- Lid lag
- Proptosis – the eye has protruded so far forward that it is visible beyond the level of the supraorbital ridge when looking over the head of the patient from behind
- Exophthalmos – both eyelids move away from the centre of the iris so that the whiteness of the sclera is visible below or all round the iris
- Chemosis – the venous and lymphatic drainage is disturbed by the protrusion of the eye and the appearance is oedematous and wrinkled
- Ophthalmoplegia

In the normal eye, the upper eyelid is halfway between the pupil and the superior limbus, while the lower eyelid is at the level of the inferior limbus

Finish your examination here

Completion

Say that you would like to:

- Ask the patient how the thyroid mass is affecting their life
- Continue to assess the patients's thyroid status by:
  - asking her a few questions (*see* Case 12)
  - listening over the thyroid for a systolic bruit over the thyroid – this is caused by a hypervascular thyroid – which is almost pathognomonic of Grave's disease
- Look at the shins for pretibial myxoedema (seen in Grave's disease – *see* Case 11)
- Test for proximal myopathy by assessing the strength of the muscles of the upper arm (seen in Grave's disease)
- Test the reflexes – supinator jerks are inverted and ankle jerks are slow-relaxing in hypothyroidism

---

J Dalrymple (1804–1852). English opthalmologist.
F. de Quervain (1868–1940). Swiss surgeon who described subacute thyroiditis with self-limiting inflammation of the gland, pathologically characterized by giant cells and granuloma, which is probably as a result of viral infection. 50% of patients may experience mild hyperthyroidism.
Hakura Hashimoto (1881–1934). Japanese surgeon who described an auto-immune thyroiditis often associated with mild hypothyroidism. The pathology is thought to be due to apoptosis induced by lymphocytes bearing Fas ligands combining with thyrocytes bearing Fas.

Notes

1. The term 'goitre' is non-specific and describes any swelling of the thyroid gland. It does not imply any pathology. It is derived from the Latin for throat (*guttur*). Goitres become visible when they are three times the normal size, so that they weigh over 50 g. Goitres can be graded according to the World Health Organization (WHO) grading scheme:

Grade 0   No palpable or visible goitre
Grade 1   Palpable goitre
Grade 1A Goitre detectable only by palpation
Grade 1B Goitre palpable and visible with neck extended
Grade 2   Goitre visible with neck in normal position
Grade 3   Large goitre visible from a distance

2. Patients with large retrosternal goitres develop signs of compression on raising their arms above their heads, leading to suffusion of the face, giddiness or syncope. This is Pemberton's sign – do not elicit in the examination as the patient may faint.

3. There are some other physical signs of the eye which are of historic interest that are included here for sake of completeness:
   – Stellwag's sign – *C. Stellwag von Carion (1823–1904), Austrian opthalmologist* – infrequent blinking in hyperthyroidism
   – Joffroy's sign – *A. Joffroy (1844–1908), French neuropsychiatrist* – absence of wrinkling of the forehead when the patient bends her head and looks up
   – Mobius' sign – *P. J. Mobius (1853–1907), German neurologist* – difficulty in convergence elicited in a patient with ophthalmoplegia

4. The term vitiligo is derived from the Latin *vitellus* for 'spotted calf'

*** SOLITARY THYROID NODULE   CASE 9

INSTRUCTION

See Cases 6 and 8 for the general examination of the neck and thyroid gland.

SPECIFIC POINTS ON EXAMINATION OF THE NECK

- Palpable nodule which moves on swallowing but not on protrusion of tongue
- Palpate for associated cervical lymphadenopathy

QUESTIONS

(a) What are the causes of a solitary thyroid nodule?

- Prominent nodule in a multinodular goitre
- Cyst (caused by haemorrhage into a necrotic nodule)
- Adenoma
- Carcinoma/lymphoma
- Thyroiditis (*see* Case 8)

(b) What do you know about solitary thyroid nodules?

- More common in females (F:M ratio = 4:1)
- Occur most commonly in the fourth and fifth decade

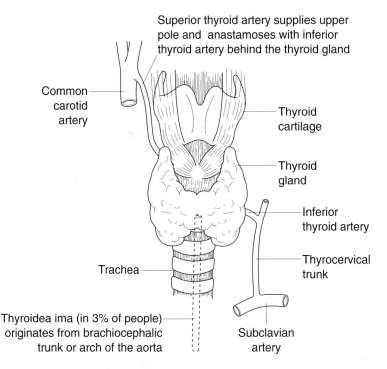

Fig. 6   Anatomy of the arterial supply to the thyroid gland.

- 10% in middle-aged are malignant *but* 50% are malignant in the young and the elderly
- Fine-needle aspiration cytology (FNAC) is the most important investigation – if benign, leave alone and if malignant, surgery is required
- Technetium radioisotope scans differentiate cold from hot nodules
- Cold nodules that are solid or partly cystic must be regarded malignant until proven otherwise

(c) How would you investigate and treat a solitary thyroid nodule?

- All patients should have a clinical examination, fine-needle aspiration cytology and a technetium radio-isotope scan
- The treatment is then dependent on the findings (Fig. 7)

(d) What do you know about thyroid adenomas?

- Almost all are follicular adenomas
- Usually 2–4 cm and encapsulated at presentation
- Indistinguishable from carcinomas on fine-needle aspiration cytology, as the presence of a capsule cannot be demonstrated
- Surgical excision is needed to confirm diagnosis

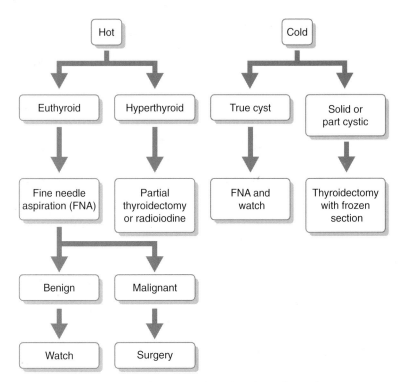

Fig. 7 Treatment algorithm for solitary thyroid nodules after radio-isotope scan.

ADVANCED QUESTIONS

(a) What do you know about thyroid malignancy?

- The incidence is low – approx 4 per 100 000 per year
- Histological varieties are:
  - papillary   = 75%
  - follicular   = 10%
  - medullary   = 8%
  - anaplastic   = 5%
  - lymphoma = 2%
- Papillary (ends in y = yellow = lymph = lymphatic spread!)
  - commonest in children and young adults
  - multicentric
  - 90% of children have nodal metastases at surgery
  - spreads to lymph nodes
  - treatment is with thyroid lobectomy or occasionally thyroidectomy
- Follicular (ends in r = red = blood = spread via bloodstream!)
  - mean age is 50 years at presentation

- FNA cannot distinguish cancer from follicular adenoma
- note that 80% of follicular lesions on FNA are adenomas
- spread via bloodstream
- treatment is total thyroidectomy and lifelong thyroxine replacement therapy +/– radioiodine to ablate residual malignant cells
- Medullary
  - arises from the parafollicular C cells (derived from ultimobranchial bodies) which produce calcitonin, a polypeptide which decreases blood calcium
  - 90% are sporadic cases
  - 10% are familial and may be associated with multiple endocrine neoplasia type II (see below)
  - familial cases are associated with mutations of the RET proto-oncogene – if mutation present, 100% risk of developing medullary carcinoma and therefore prophylactic thyroidectomy is indicated in childhoood
  - treatment is radical surgery with follow-up using sequential calcitonin assays
- Anaplastic
  - occur in the elderly
  - debulking is the only possible option
  - treatment with radiotherapy and doxorubicin gives best survival of 1 year
- Lymphoma
  - trucut biopsy is often needed for diagnosis
  - treated with radiotherapy and chemotherapy

(b) What do you know about thyroid cysts?

- True cysts with a completely smooth wall are very rare
- Most are composite lesions with colloid degeneration, necrosis or haemorrhage in benign or malignant tumours
- Only benign if *completely* abolished by aspiration
- Note that cytology can be false-negative in a third of malignant cysts

Notes

Multiple endocrine neoplasia type I (Wermer syndrome):

- Autosomal dominant
- **P**ancreatic islet cell tumour
- **P**ituitary adenoma
- **P**rimary hyperparathyroidism

Multiple endocrine neoplasia type IIa (Sipple syndrome):

- Autosomal dominant
- Phaeochromocytoma
- Medullary carcinoma of the thyroid
- Primary hyperparathyroidism

Multiple endocrine neoplasia type IIb:
- Same as IIa but no parathyroid involvement

J. H. Sipple (1930–). North American Professor of Medicine, New York
P. Wermer. Contemporary North American physician, Columbia University, New York

FURTHER READING

Walsh R M, Watkinson J C and Franklyn J (1999) The management of the solitary thyroid nodule: a review. *Clin Otolaryngol* **24**(5): 388–97.

*** **MULTINODULAR GOITRE**   **CASE 10**

INSTRUCTION

See Cases 6 and 8 for the general examination of the neck and thyroid gland.

SPECIFIC POINTS ON EXAMINATION OF THE NECK

With a large multinodular goitre it should be relatively easy to palpate the thyroid as the patient swallows some water:
- Describe the features of the lump:
  - multinodular
  - may be large in size
  - there may be one nodule which is more prominent than the others
- Check the position of the trachea, which may be deviated by a large multinodular goitre, and percuss for retrosternal extension

OTHER POINTS ON SYSTEMIC EXAMINATION

- Feel the pulse – atrial fibrillation is seen in 40% of patients with multinodular goitre

QUESTIONS

(a) What are the features of a multinodular goitre (MNG)?

- Progression of simple diffuse goitre to nodular enlargement
- Middle-aged women
- Positive family history. Malignant change occurs in 5% of untreated MNGs
- Overactivity in parts of an MNG may lead to mild hyperthyroidism (Plummer's Syndrome)
- No ophthalmic features are seen (these are characteristic of Grave's disease – case 11)

(b) How would you manage a multinodular goitre?

- After taking a history and performing a clinical examination, most patients do not need any intervention
- The patient usually presents because of:
  - cosmetic reasons, or they have noticed a lump in their neck
  - discomfort
  - tracheal compression – causing shortness of breath
  - oesophageal compression – causing dysphagia
  - worries about malignancy
  - onset of hyperthyroidism
- Investigate if:
  - prominent nodule
  - features suspicious of malignancy, such as cervical lymphadenopathy or recurrent laryngeal nerve palsy
- Investigate using:
  - thyroid function tests – hyperthyroid?
  - ultrasound – dimensions of goitre and nodules, look for cysts that can be aspirated
  - chest X-ray – a retrosternal goitre may compress the trachea
  - technetium scintiscan – demonstrates hyperfunctioning and cold nodules
  - fine-needle aspiration cytology – especially cold nodules

(c) How would you treat a multinodular goitre?

- Non-surgical:
  - remove goitrogens, e.g. remove cabbage from diet
  - thyroxine 0.1–0.3 mg per day – causes regression in 50–70% of patients probably because multinodular goitres increase in size as a result of raised thyroid-stimulating hormone levels
  - if thyrotoxicosis, treat as in Grave's disease (*see* Case 11)
  - aspiration of cysts with cytology to exclude malignancy, and treat recurrent simple cysts with instillation of tetracycline
  - radioiodine – for elderly patients, particularly those unfit for surgery
- Surgical:
  - bilateral subtotal thyroidectomy with postoperative replacement of thyroxine
  - avoid total thyroidectomy due to risk of damage to recurrent laryngeal nerve and parathyroids, although some surgeons do prefer a total thyroidectomy with careful preservation of the laryngeal nerves and the parathyroid glands

(d) What are the indications for surgery?

- Obstructive symptoms
- Suspicion of malignancy
- Cosmetic reasons
- Thyrotoxicosis
- Increasing size despite adequate thyroxine therapy
- Retrosternal extension

ADVANCED QUESTIONS

(a) How can you tell the difference between toxic multinodular goitre and Grave's disease?

See Table 3.

Table 3

Toxic multinodular goitre	Grave's disease
Older age group	Younger age-group
Nodular enlargement	Diffuse enlargement
Eye signs not present	Eye signs present
Atrial fibrillation present in 40% of patients	Atrial fibrillation uncommon
No associated autoimmune diseases	Autoimmune diseases commonly associated

---

H. S. Plummer (1874–1936). North American physician. Also described:

- Plummer nails – concave or ragged edge to the nail-bed seen in early onycholysis occurring in thyrotoxicosis (most prominent in fourth and fifth fingers)
- Plummer sign – inability of patient to sit in a chair as a result of thyrotoxic myopathy
- Plummer treatment – the use of iodine to treat thyrotoxicosis
- Plummer–Vinson syndrome – iron deficiency anaemia associated with dysphagia and post-cricoid oesophageal webs in middle-aged women (note that this is the North American variation – this syndrome is known as the Paterson-Brown-Kelly syndrome in the United Kingdom and the Waldenstrom-Kjellberg syndrome in Scandinavia!)

FURTHER READING

Hisham A N, Azlina A F, Aina E N, Sarojah A (2001) Total thyroidectomy: the procedure of choice for multinodular goitre. *Eur J Surg* **6**: 403–5.

Huysmans D, Hermus A, Edelbroek M, Barentsz J, Corstens F, Kloppenborg P (1997) Radioiodine for nontoxic multinodular goitre. *Thyroid* **7**(2): 235–9.

CASE 11   DIFFUSE THYROID ENLARGEMENT   ***

INSTRUCTION

See Cases 6 and 8 for the general examination of the neck and thyroid gland.

SPECIFIC POINTS ON EXAMINATION OF THE NECK

- Describe the features of the lump:
  - diffuse enlargement (not nodular)
  - may be large in size
  - non-tender
- Gently palpate the trachea for deviation (from a large goitre), and ask the patient if she has had any problems swallowing (from a large goitre) or noticed any change in her voice
- Remember to percuss over the sternum for a retrosternal extension of a large goitre

QUESTIONS

(a) What are the causes of a diffusely enlarged thyroid gland?

- Simple colloid goitre
- Grave's disease
- Thyroiditis (Hashimoto's, de Quervain's or Riedels's – *see* Case 8)

(b) What do you know about simple colloid goitres?

- Commonest form of thyroid abnormality
- Secondary to hyperplasia of the gland to meet physiological demand for thyroxine
- Secondary to defective production of thyroid hormone
- Causes are as follows:
  - iodine deficiency – commonest cause worldwide
  - increased physiological demand -puberty, pregnancy and lactation (commonest cause in the UK)
  - goitrogens (less common) – uncooked cabbage, lithium and anti-thyroid drugs
  - defects of thyroid hormone production (rare)

(c) What are the features of Grave's disease?

- Commoner in females (9:1)
- Results from polyclonal immunoglobulins against thyroid-stimulating hormone receptor which bind and stimulate the receptor – these antibodies are found in 90% of patients
- Hyperthyroidism with goitre

- Thyroid eye disease (*see* Case 8)
- Thyroid acropachy
- Pretibial myxoedema
- Normochromic normocytic anaemia, raised erythrocyte sedimentation rate and hypercalcaemia can also occur
- Associated with other autoimmune conditions such as Type 1 diabetes and pernicious anaemia

(d) How do you treat Grave's disease?

- Medical:
  - antithyroid drugs, e.g. carbimazole, methimazole, propylthiouracil – to inhibit thyroid peroxidase
  - beta-blockers, e.g. propanolol – to reduce the effects of excess circulating thyroxine on the cardiac system
- Radioiodine:
  - treatment of choice (only absolute contraindications are pregnancy and lactation)
  - single oral dose of ^{131}I causes direct radiation damage to the replication mechanisms of thyroid follicular cells
  - risks include early hyperthyroidism, late hypothyroidism and late hyperparathyroidism
- Surgery:
  - bilateral subtotal thyroidectomy leaving behind 4–10 g of thyroid tissue
  - particularly useful for: patients who refuse radiation therapy, pregnant patients or those wishing to become pregnant within 4 years, patients under the age of 30 years and those with nodular or large goitres

(e) What are the complications of thyroidectomy?

Complications of thyroidectomy can be divided into those that are general to any operation (e.g. risks of anaesthesia) and those that are specific to thyroidectomy alone. They can also be divided into *immediate* (within 24 hours), *early* (within 30 days) and *late* (after 30 days) – they (mostly) begin with the letter H:

- Immediate:
  - **H**aemorrhage, leading to airway obstruction from secondary laryngeal oedema; patients who have recently had a thyroid operation should have a pair of suture cutters by their bed – if this complication occurs the sutures should immediately be removed and an anaesthetist called
  - **H**oarseness from damage to the recurrent laryngeal nerve
  - **H**yperthyroidism – severe and is known as thyroid storm
- Early:
  - (**H**)infection – a rather weak H!
  - **H**ypoparathyroidism, leading to **H**ypocalcaemia
- Late:
  - **H**yperthyroidism – recurrent
  - **H**ypothyroidism
  - **H**ypertrophic scarring

ADVANCED QUESTIONS

(a) What is the pathology of thyroid eye disease?

- Exophthalmos is secondary to retrorbital inflammation and lymphocytic infiltration, leading to oedema and an increase in retrobulbar orbital contents
- Lid lag is secondary to sympathetic overstimulation and restrictive myopathy of levator palpebrae superioris

(b) How do you classify the severity of thyroid eye disease?

Use Werner's mnemonic **NO SPECS** (Table 4)

Table 4 NO SPECS **classification of thyroid eye disease**

Class 0	**N**	**N**o signs or symptoms
Class 1	**O**	**O**nly signs of upper lid retraction and stare, with or without lid lag and exophthalmos
Class 2	**S**	**S**oft-tissue involvement
Class 3	**P**	**P**roptosis
Class 4	**E**	**E**xophthalmos
Class 5	**C**	**C**orneal involvement
Class 6	**S**	**S**ight loss due to optic nerve involvement

R. J. Graves (1797–1853). Irish physician, Dublin

FURTHER READING

Weetman A P (2000) Graves' disease. *N Engl J Med.* **343**(17): 236–48.

INSTRUCTION

This lady is complaining of a swelling in her neck. Ask her a few questions about her thyroid gland.

APPROACH

It is important to ascertain the symptoms arising from the swelling, the thyroid status, other associated symptoms and any relevant medical history:

Symptoms arising from the swelling

- Duration and change in size – note particularly if the swelling has suddenly increased in size (can occur if there is haemorrhage into a necrotic nodule, subacute thyroiditis or a rapidly growing carcinoma)
- Cosmetic symptoms
- Discomfort during swallowing/dysphagia – oesophageal compression
- Dyspnoea (tracheal compression)
- Hoarseness – due to recurrent laryngeal nerve paralysis secondary to malignant infiltration
- Pain – not common but can occur in thyroiditis or anaplastic carcinoma

Thyroid status

Table 5 shows the symptoms of hyper- and hypothyroidism.

Other associated symptoms

- Ask about eye symptoms, e.g. protruding or staring eyes, difficulty closing eyelids, double vision (secondary to ophthalmoplegia) and pain in the eye (secondary to corneal ulceration)

Relevant medical history

- Previous operations on the thyroid gland
- Previous or current medication, e.g. antithyroid drugs, thyroxine, iodine-containing medications
- Radioiodine therapy for previous Grave's disease (eye signs may persist)
- Move on to assessing fitness for surgery if relevant and time permits

Table 5

	Hyperthyroidism	Hypothyroidism
General	Increased appetite but loss of weight	Decreased appetite and gain in weight, lethargy
Thermoregulatory	Preference for cold weather	Preference for hot weather
Dermatological	Increased sweating	Dry skin, 'peaches and cream' complexion, loss of hair – especially outer third of eyebrows
Musculoskeletal	Proximal myopathy (autoimmune) with wasting and weakness	Muscle fatigue
Gastrointestinal	Change in bowel habit, particularly diarrhoea and frequent defaecation	Constipation
Cardiovascular	Tachycardia, atrial fibrillation	Bradycardia
Gynaecological	Oligomenorrhoea, amenorrhoea	Menorrhagia
Psychiatric	Nervousness, easy irritability, emotional lability, insomnia; psychosis	Slow thought, speech and action, depression, dementia
Neurological	Fine tremor	Symptoms of carpal tunnel syndrome (see Case 79)

INSTRUCTION

No specific instruction other than being asked to inspect the scar.

APPROACH

Your description is likely to be based solely on inspection.

VITAL POINTS

- The scar can be on any part of the body where there has been an incision in the skin
- Describe the scar – point out that the scar area is more prominent than the surrounding skin and add details as in Table 6

Table 6

Features	Hypertrophic scars	Keloid scars
Appearance	Scar confined to wound margins	Scar extends beyond wound margins
Site	Across flexor surfaces and skin creases	Earlobes, chin, neck, shoulder, chest

Finish your examination here

Completion

Say that you would like to:
- Ask the patient how the scar affects their lives, e.g. cosmetic symptoms, pain and itching

QUESTIONS

(a) What do you know about the epidemiology of hypertrophic and keloid scars?

See Table 7.

Table 7

Features	Hypertrophic scars	Keloid scars
Age	Any age (commonly 8–20 years)	Puberty to 30 years
Gender	M = F	F > M
Race	All races	Black and Hispanic races

(b) What types of wounds are prone to hypertrophic and keloid scar formation?

Wounds associated with:
- Infection
- Trauma
- Burns
- Tension, especially over the sternum such as after coronary artery bypass grafting
- Wounds on certain areas of the body, see Table 6

(c) Is there a difference in the clinical course of hypertrophic and keloid scars?

Hypertrophic scars tend to appear soon after injury and usually regress spontaneously, while keloid scars appear months after injury and continue to grow.

(d) How do you treat these scars?

Recurrence can be as high as 55% with surgical revision alone, and therefore a combination of the treatments outlined below is often employed:

- Non-surgical – mechanical pressure therapy (day and night for up to a year), topical silicone gel sheets
- Surgical – revision of scar with closure by direct suturing, local Z-plasty or skin grafting to avoid excessive tension
- Intralesional steroid and local anaesthetic injections – using triamcinolone in combination with lignocaine

ADVANCED QUESTIONS

(a) What other associations have been described with keloid and hypertrophic scars?

See Table 8.

Table 8

Associations	Hypertrophic scars	Keloid scars
Biochemical	Normal rate of collagen synthesis but increased breakdown of collagen by collagenase activity	Increased rate of collagen synthesis (increased proline hydroxylase activity) and increased collagenase activity
Genetic	Not proven	Significant predisposition in Black and Hispanic races
Oxygen levels	Relative hypoxia – due to wound tension?	No link
Immunology	May be important, but no specific associations known	Increased IgG, IgM and C3 levels, and antinuclear antibodies to keloid fibroblasts

FURTHER READING

English R S, Shenefelt P D (1999) Keloids and hypertrophic scars. *Dermatol Surg* **25**(8): 631–8.

> *Jean Louis Albert* coined the name 'keloid' in 1806 in order to describe this 'overhealing' phenomenon, although they had been originally described in the Smith Surgical Papyrus (2500 BC).

*** SQUAMOUS CELL CARCINOMA CASE 14

INSTRUCTION

'Examine this gentleman's face.'

APPROACH

Sit or kneel in front of the patient in order to be at the same level as his face, and examine as for any lump.

VITAL POINTS

Inspect

- May occur on any part of the face (usually in areas of sun-exposed skin where skin looks 'weathered')
- Appears vascular (red-brown)
- Raised and everted edge
- May be of considerable size (> 1 cm)
- There may be erosion of the facial architecture if the tumour is advanced
- May have central ulceration

Palpate

- Regional cervical lymphadenopathy (may be due to metastases or secondary infection – only 5% have metastasized by the time of presentation) (*see* Case 6)

Finish your examination here

Completion

Say that you would like to:

- Ask the patient about predisposing factors (see below)
- How the lesion affects his life, e.g. cosmetic symptoms

QUESTIONS

(a) What is your differential diagnosis?

Benign skin lesions:

- Keratoacanthoma
- Infected seborrhoeic wart
- Solar keratosis
- Pyogenic granuloma

Malignant skin lesions:

- Basal cell carcinoma
- Malignant melanoma (amelanotic)

(b) What are the predisposing factors for squamous cell carcinomas (SCC)?

Congenital:

- Xeroderma pigmentosum (*see* Case 16)

Acquired:

- Environmental agents, e.g. sunlight, ionizing radiation, industrial carcinogens such as arsenic
- Pre-existing skin lesions, e.g. solar keratosis (*see* Case 27), Bowen's disease (see below)
- Infections, e.g. viral warts (human papilloma virus 5 and 8)
- Immunosuppression, e.g. in anti-rejection treatment post-transplant and in HIV infection – may develop multiple SCCs
- Chronic cutaneous ulceration, e.g. chronic burns, chronic venous ulcers (Marjolin's ulcer)

(c) What treatment options are available for SCC?

Primary lesion:

- Excision with 1 cm margin
- Moh's staged chemosurgery with histological assessment of margins and electrodessication – for lesions of the eyelids, ears and nasolabial folds
- Radiotherapy – for unresectable lesions

Nodal spread:

- Surgical block dissection – if palpable nodes or in cases of Marjolin's ulcers but the benefit of prophylactic block lymph node dissection with Marjolin's ulcers is not proven
- Radiotherapy

ADVANCED QUESTIONS

(a) What do you know about the pathology of SCC?

The tumour arises from epidermal cells that normally migrate to the skin surface to form the superficial keratinising squamous layer. Full-thickness epidermal atypia is seen (versus basal atypia only in solar keratosis) and tumour cells are seen to extend in all directions into the deep dermis and subcutaneous fat. The tumour itself may be well differentiated (with production of keratin), moderately differentiated or poorly differentiated.

Professor J. T. Bowen (1857–1941). American dermatologist. Bowen's disease is an intraepidermal carcinoma presenting as a single brown-red irregular plaque usually on the trunk that increases in size and may progress to invasive SCC. The condition is also associated with subsequent development of visceral malignancies, usually 5–7 years later, particularly if the affected area of skin has never been exposed to the sun. Excision with at least a 0.5 cm margin is recommended. When seen on the penis, vulva or oral cavity, it is known as *Erythroplasia of Queyrat* (French dermatologist c.1900)
R. Marjolin (1812–1895). French surgeon

FURTHER READING

Goldman G D (1998) Squamous cell cancer: a practical approach. *Semin Cutan Med Surg* **17**(2): 80–95.

http://www.scfa.edu.au/scc.html – general information about SCCs.

*** MALIGNANT MELANOMA CASE 15

INSTRUCTION

'Examine the lesion on this lady's right leg. What do you think it is?'

APPROACH

The patient should already be adequately exposed. Examine as for any lump (*see* Case 1).

VITAL POINTS

Inspect

- Found most commonly on the legs of young women and the trunk of middle-aged men, but location and characteristics depend on type

- Commonest cancer of young adults aged between 20 and 39 years
- Commoner in women than men

The four commonest types are:

Superficial spreading melanoma
- Most common type (70%)
- Occurs most often on the legs of women and the backs of men
- Red, white and blue in colour
- Irregular edge
- Usually palpable but thin

Nodular melanoma
- Second most common type (15–30%)
- Occurs most often on the trunk
- Polypoid in shape and is raised
- Smooth surface
- Irregular edge
- Frequently ulcerated

Lentigo maligna melanoma
- Arises in a lentigo maligna (Hutchinson's melanotic freckle – see below)
- Occurs most often on the face or dorsum of the hands and forearms
- Underlying lesion is flat and brown-to-black in colour with an irregular outline
- Malignant area in the lesion is usually thicker, and darker in colour

Acral lentiginous melanoma
- Least common
- Occurs on hairless skin (such as subungual area, and palms of hands and soles and feet), and is more common in Oriental and Black races
- Irregular area of brown or black pigmentation

There are other more rare types of melanoma (e.g. amelanotic melanoma with no pigmentation and a poorer prognosis) but these are less likely to be encountered in the clinical cases. It is also possible to have intra-cranial melanoma as there is melanin in the substantia nigra, and also in the retina.

Features of a pigmented skin lesion suspicious of malignancy

- Loss of normal surface markings around the lesion (e.g. skin creases)
- Presence of ulceration
- Evidence of bleeding from the lesion
- Marked variation of colour within the lesion
- Presence of a halo of brown pigment in the skin around the lesion
- Presence of satellite nodules of tumour around the lesion

Finish your examination here

Completion

Say that you would like to:

- Examine the draining lymph nodes

- Ask the patient about symptoms from the lesion that may indicate malignancy, e.g. rapid increase in the size of a mole, itching, bleeding, change in colour, shape or thickness
- Ask the patient about predisposing factors (see below)

QUESTIONS

(a) What is your differential diagnosis?

Benign skin lesions:

- Moles – increased numbers of melanocytes producing too much melanin (also called pigmented naevus)
- Freckles – normal numbers of melanocytes but each producing too much melanin
- Lentigo – increased numbers of melanocytes producing normal amounts of melanin
- Pigmented seborrhoeic keratoses
- Dermatofibromas (*see* Case 33)
- Thrombosed haemangiomas

Malignant skin lesions:

- Pigmented basal cell carcinomas (*see* Case 16)

(b) What are the predisposing factors for malignant melanomas?

Congenital:

- Xeroderma pigmentosum (*see* Case 16)
- Dysplastic naevus syndrome (also known as B-K mole or FAMM syndrome) – risk of developing malignant melanoma is 100% if two family members are affected
- Large congenital naevi
- Family history in first-degree relatives (increased risk by one and a half times)

Acquired:

- Sunlight (particularly ultraviolet light) – especially in fair-skinned people with red hair
- Pre-existing skin lesions, e.g. lentigo maligna, more than 20 benign pigmented naevi (the latter increases the risk three times)
- Previous melanoma (increases the risk three and a half times)

(c) How do you stage malignant melanomas?

There are two pathological staging systems in use, both of which have prognostic value. Both staging systems are based on the depth of invasion of the tumour from the epidermis. The first is Clark's levels of invasion (Fig. 8), described in 1969 (Table 9).

Table 9

Clark's level	Extent of tumour	5-year survival
I	Epidermis only	98%
II	Invades papillary dermis	96%
III	Fills papillary dermis	94%
IV	Invades reticular dermis	78%
V	Subcutaneous tissue invasion	44%

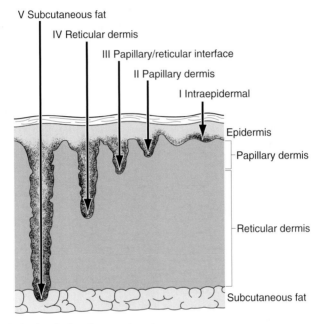

Fig. 8 Clark's level of melanoma invasion.

The second is Breslow's thickness (Fig. 9), described in 1970 (Table 10).

Table 10

Breslow thickness	10-year survival
< 0.76 mm	92%
< 3 mm	50%
< 4 mm	30%
Lymph node involvement	< 40% (8-year survival)

Breslow's thickness is a better prognostic indicator because the reticular dermis is not uniformly thick in different parts of the body.

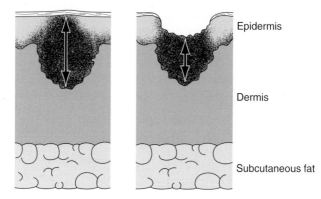

Fig. 9 Breslow's thickness of malignant melanoma, which relates to thickness of the tumour itself.

A four-stage clinically based system is also in use, which is more accurate for prognosis (Beahrs and Myers 1983) (Table 11).

Table 11

Clinical stage	Histopathological stage
IA	< 0.75 mm or Clark level II
IB	0.75–1.5 mm or Clark level III
IIA	1.5–4.0 mm or Clark level IV
IIB	> 4.0 mm or Clark level V
III	Lymph node metastasis in one regional drainage area, or > 5 in transit metastasis
IV	Advanced regional metastasis or distant metastasis

(d) What treatment options are available for malignant melanoma?

Surgical excision

Main lesion:

Veronesi has been instrumental in leading opinion as to the most appropriate surgical management of melanoma:

- Lesions < 0.76 mm – excise with a 1 cm margin of grossly normal tissue
- Lesions 0.76–1.0 mm – excise with a 2 cm margin
- Lesions > 1.0 mm – excise with a 3 cm margin
- Excision should be down to deep fascia

Nodal spread:
- If clinical suspicion of nodal metastasis, lymph node biopsy or fine-needle aspiration cytology (FNAC)
- If palpable lymph nodes, therapeutic block dissection

Palliation/adjuvant therapies for distant metastases
- Intralesional BCG therapy
- Immunotherapy, e.g. vaccines to raise an anti-melanoma antibody response, monoclonal antibody therapy, cytokine interferon therapy

Prevention – MOST IMPORTANT to mention this in your answer
- Avoidance of causative factors, e.g. public education campaigns to reduce sun exposure

ADVANCED QUESTIONS

(a) What do you know about the pathology of malignant melanoma?

On microscopy, malignant melanomas consist of loose nests of melanocytes in the basal cell layer which invade the epidermis (leading to destruction and ulceration) and penetrate deeper into the dermis and subcutaneous fat.

(b) Do you know of any prognostic indicators for malignant melanoma?

Clark's levels, Breslow's thickness and the four-stage clinical system have been described above. In addition, the following are also known to be indicators of poor prognosis:

- Increasing age of the patient
- Male patients
- Melanomas on the trunk (especially the back), scalp, hand and foot
- Ulceration of the tumour
- Depigmentation and amelanotic melanomas
- Aneuploidy and high mitotic index

Sir John Hunter (1728–1793). First described malignant melanoma in 1787. *See* Case 117.

Sir Jonathan Hutchinson (1828–1913). English surgeon, London Hospital and Professor of Surgery, Royal College of Surgeons. He described a flat pigmented, brown-to-black melanocytic naevus with malignant potential that occurs on sun-damaged skin on the face, and on the dorsum of the hands and forearm. The freckle itself represents an increased number of melanocytes at the dermoepidermal junction. It occurs in the fifth to seventh decades, and after a period of time (10–30 years), it transforms into a malignant melanoma, heralded clinically by the development of a black or tan nodule. Also described Hutchinson triad (eighth nerve deafness, notched teeth and interstitial keratitis in congenital syphilis).

FURTHER READING

Reintgen D, Cruse C W, Atkins M (2001) Cutaneous malignant melanoma. *Clin Dermatol* **19**(3): 253–61.

Beahrs O H, Myers M H (1983) Manual for Staging of Cancer. *Am Joint Comm Cancer*. Philadelphia, Lippincott: 117.

http://www.skincancerfacts.org.uk – information on all types of skin cancers for patients.

** BASAL CELL CARCINOMA CASE 16

INSTRUCTION

'Examine this gentleman's face.'

APPROACH

Sit or kneel in front of the patient in order to be at the same level as his face, and examine as for any lump.

VITAL POINTS

> TOP TIP
> If you need to see the side of the patient's face, e.g. ear, stay still while sitting or kneeling and ask the patient to turn his head to the appropriate side – it looks unprofessional to keep darting around the patient!

Inspect

- Occur on hair-bearing sun-exposed skin of elderly people, especially around the eye
- Single or multiple
- Features of basal cell carcinomata (BCCs) depend on the clinical type and can be divided into:

Raised above the skin

- Nodular/nodulo-ulcerative
  - most common type
  - well-defined rolled, pearly edge
  - central ulceration
- Cystic
  - large cystic nodule

Not raised above the skin

- Pigmented
  - contains melanin
  - can be confused with malignant melanoma (*see* Case 15)
- Sclerosing (also known as morphoeic)
  - flat or depressed tumour
  - ill-defined edge
  - may be ulcerated (occurs late)
- Cicatricial (also known as field-fire or bush-fire)
  - multiple superficial erythematous lesions interspersed with pale atrophic areas
- Superficial
  - erythematous scaly patches
  - can be confused with Bowen's disease (*see* Case 14)

Palpate

- Fixation of the BCC deep to the skin is a sign of deep local invasion

Finish your examination here

Completion

Say that you would like to:

- Examine for regional lymphadenopathy (but note that metastases are extremely rare, BCCs are locally aggressive)
- Ask the patient about predisposing factors (see below)

QUESTIONS

(a) What is your differential diagnosis?

The two main differential diagnoses to consider are:

- Benign – keratoacanthoma – especially if it is sloughing at its centre (*see* Case 22)
- Malignant – squamous cell carcinoma – particularly the nodulo-ulcerative type with a rolled edge (*see* Case 14)

(b) What are the predisposing factors for basal cell carcinomas (BCC)?

- Congenital (rare):
  - xeroderma pigmentosum (familial condition associated with failure of DNA transcription, leading to defective DNA repair) – also known as Kaposi's disease (*see* Cases 16 and 35)
  - Gorlin's syndrome (see below)
- Acquired (very common):
  - sunlight (particularly ultraviolet light in the UVB range)
  - carcinogens, e.g. cigarette smoke, arsenic
  - previous radiotherapy
  - malignant transformation in pre-existing skin lesions, e.g. naevus sebaceous

(c) What treatment options are available for BCC?

Treatment options available are:

- Tumours raised above the skin – excision with 0.5 cm margin (maximum)
- Tumours not raised above the skin – wider margin of excision, particularly if at inner canthus of eye, nasolabial fold, nasal floor and ear – frozen section may be necessary to ensure adequate excision
- Other approaches – radiotherapy and Mohs' surgery (*see* Case 14)

ADVANCED QUESTIONS

(a) What do you know about the histology of BCC?

On microscopy, BCCs have many patterns but the most common features are islands and nests of basaloid cells in the dermis (like those seen in the basal cell layer of the epidermis). The cells exhibit high mitotic rates and peripheral palisading (cell islands arranged radially with long axes in approximately parallel alignment). Often, there is ulceration of the epidermis.

(b) What do you know of the pathology of BCC?

The Hedgehog signalling pathway is important in embryological development and is highly conserved through evolution. Recently Patched, a member of the pathway, was found to be important in Gorlin's syndrome. Inherited Patched gene mutations underlie the syndrome, in which a key feature is multiple basal cell carcinomas (BCCs). The gene is also mutated in sporadic BCCs.

> *R. J. Gorlin (1923–).* American Professor of Oral Pathology, University of Minnesota. Gorlin's syndrome (naevoid basal cell epithelioma syndrome) is an autosomal dominant condition presenting in early adult life with multiple basal cell carcinomas, keratocysts of the jaw, palmar and plantar pits, mesenteric cysts and scoliosis.

FURTHER READING

Lim J K, Stewart M M, Pennington DG (1992) Microscopically controlled excision of skin cancer. *Med J Aust* **6** 156(7): 486–8.

Gorlin R J (1995) Nevoid basal cell carcinoma syndrome. *Dermatol Clin* **13**(1): 113–25.

Saldanha G (2001) The Hedgehog signalling pathway and cancer. *J Pathol* **193**(4): 427–32.

http://www.skincancerfacts.org.uk/– information for patients on all skin cancers, including BCCs.

CASE 17   PRESSURE SORES   **

INSTRUCTION

'Have a look at this lady's heel.'

APPROACH

Examine as for ulcers (*see* Case 110). It is important to bear in mind when examining the peripheral vascular system of patients in the circulatory bay that ulcers may be due to pressure necrosis as well as peripheral vascular disease.

VITAL POINTS ON INSPECTION

You should be able to pick up all of the points simply from inspection. The American National Pressure Ulcer Advisory Panel classification should be kept in mind when describing your findings:

> TOP TIP – CLASSIFICATION OF PRESSURE SORES
> Stage 1 – Abnormal area of skin with erythema that will not blanch – indicates extravasated blood from cutaneous capillary beds
> Stage 2 – Partial thickness skin loss – a shallow abrasion wound
> Stage 3 – Full thickness skin loss with fat at the base of the wound
> Stage 4 – Extensive soft-tissue loss through deep fascia, often with underlying muscle necrosis

Completion

- Say that you would like to take a history looking for predisposing factors (see below)

QUESTIONS

(a) Where are pressure sores most commonly found?

Pressure sores can occur over any bony prominence, the commonest areas being:

- Sacrum
- Greater trochanter
- Heel
- Lateral malleolus
- Ischial tuberosity
- Occiput

(b) What conditions increase the risk of developing pressure sores?

Immobility and prolonged bed-rest are the most important factors, particularly secondary to conditions such as:

- Cardiopulmonary disease
- Trauma

- Neurological disease, e.g. paraplegia
- Bone and joint disease
- Prolonged operative procedures, particularly if there are intraoperative episodes of hypotension

Conditions that slow wound healing can increase the severity and risk of pressure necrosis:

- Metabolic disorders:
  – diabetes mellitus
  – deficiencies of vitamins and trace metals, e.g. vitamin C, zinc
- Drugs:
  – steroids
  – post-chemotherapy (also radiotherapy)
- Underlying disease:
  – tissue hypoxia such as in peripheral vascular disease
  – renal failure
  – jaundice
  – carcinomatosis
  – infection

ADVANCED QUESTIONS

(a) How do you treat this condition?

- Prophylaxis – regular skin inspection, frequent turning of immobile patients (2–4-hourly), massage, toileting, the use of special mattresses and cushions which redistribute the pressure on at-risk areas
- Non-surgical – optimize tissue perfusion and oxygenation, treat infection as it arises, use various topical dressings as required and provide nutritional support. Specifically, vitamin C, zinc and multivitamins should be prescribed. Several other techniques such as hyperbaric oxygen, hydrotherapy and ultrasound are in use depending on local policy
- Surgical – debridement of dead tissue (which often does not require anaesthesia and can be performed by the tissue viability nurse) and reconstruction using a variety of fascial and muscle-containing composite flaps, e.g. buttock rotation flap for sacral sores

(b) What do you know about the pathophysiology of pressure necrosis?

Prolonged weight-bearing and mechanical shear forces act on areas of soft-tissue overlying bony prominences, leading to both occlusion and tearing of small blood vessels, reduced tissue perfusion and ischaemic necrosis.

FURTHER READING

Cervo F A, Cruz A C, and Posillico J A (2000). Pressure ulcers. Analysis of guidelines for treatment and management. *Geriatrics* **55**(3): 55–60.

CASE 18   GRAFTS AND FLAPS   **

INSTRUCTION

You may be shown a patient who has had an operation involving a skin graft or a flap. It is important to be aware of the principles involved and the various types of grafts and flaps that may be encountered.

QUESTIONS

(a) What is a skin graft?

A skin graft involves the transfer of skin from a donor site to a recipient site independent of a blood supply. The graft 'takes' by acquiring a blood supply from a healthy donor bed. Skin grafts may either be full thickness or partial thickness, but contain the entire epidermis, with a portion of the underlying dermis. The dermis does not regenerate, but the epidermis regenerates from the 'adnexal elements of skin' – hair follicles, sebaceous glands and sweat glands within the dermis.

(b) What tissues do skin grafts not take on?

- Unhealthy, necrotic and infected tissue
- Irradiated tissue
- Exposed cortical bone without periosteum
- Tendon without peritenon
- Cartilage without perichondrium

(c) How do you harvest a skin graft?

- Use hand-held skin graft knives (e.g. Watson and Braithwaite modifications of the Humby knife) or electric- or gas-powered dermatomes, the latter producing a graft of even thickness from almost any site, with little expertise needed for operation
- Donor site is usually one that can be easily concealed, e.g. inner thigh, buttock or inner arm

(d) What is a skin flap?

A skin flap consists of tissue, or tissues, transferred from one site of the body to another, while maintaining a continuous blood supply through a vascular pedicle.

(e) How do you classify skin flaps?

- Site – local or distant (also known as a 'free flap')
- Contents – can contain any tissue capable of transfer, including omentum and bowel
- Random or axial – the latter is based on a named artery or vein

(f) What are the indications for flap reconstruction?

- Situations where skin grafts will not take (see above)
- When the aim is to reconstruct with tissue that is 'like-for-like' (bone, joint, tendon, nerve, epithelial lining, etc) to promote optimal structure, function and cosmesis
- When blood supply has to be imported to areas of doubtful viability, e.g. pressure sores, complex trauma

(g) What is the 'reconstruction ladder'?

This is the array of plastic surgical reconstruction techniques of increasing complexity, that is available to the surgeon and which are used according to their suitability for individual patients:

- Healing by secondary intention (i.e. granulation) and then by primary intention (excision and closure) prior to reconstruction
- Skin graft
- Local flap
- Distant flap
- Composite flap
- Island flaps versus pedicled flaps
- Free tissue transfer
- Composite neurovascular free tissue transfer

FURTHER READING

Valencia I C, Falabella A, Eaglstein W H (2000) Skin grafting. *Dermatol Clin* **18**(3): 521–32.

** PTOSIS   CASE 19

INSTRUCTION

'Examine this gentleman's face and tell me your diagnosis.'

APPROACH

This case is likely to be a spot diagnosis. Remember that the definition of ptosis is drooping of the upper eyelid associated with the inability to elevate the eyelid completely.

VITAL POINTS

Ptosis is best observed with the patient sitting up and the head being held by the candidate.

TOP TIP
- The upper eyelid is raised by the action of levator palpebrae superioris. This muscle is of dual origin and innervation (and is a favourite of surgical examiners):
  - mainly skeletal muscle innervated by the third cranial nerve (oculomotor)
  - a thin sheet of smooth muscle (Muller's muscle) that is supplied by postganglionic sympathetic nerve fibres arising from cell bodies in the superior cervical ganglion
- Complete ptosis follows third nerve palsy – the eyelid droops in all positions
- Partial ptosis follows an ipsilateral sympathetic nerve lesion – this is Horner's syndrome (ptosis, meiosis, anhydrosis and enophthalmos), which can be overcome on asking the patient to look up.

Inspect

- Is it unilateral or bilateral?
- Note whether ptosis is partial or complete by asking the patient to look upwards
- Look at the size of the pupil
  - small pupil in Horner's syndrome (look for other signs of Horner's – see above)
  - large pupil in third cranial nerve palsy (look at the position of the eye – down and out in third nerve palsy) and test the reaction of the pupil to light and accommodation – pupil does not react in third nerve palsy

Finish your examination here

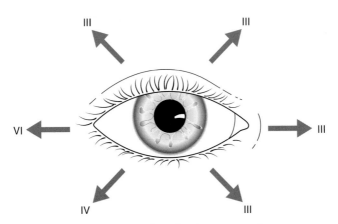

Fig. 10   The actions of the IIIrd, IVth and VIth nerves on the eye movements of the RIGHT eye. III = oculomotor, IV = trochlear, VI = abducent.

Completion

Say that you would like to take a history from the patient to try to find the cause of their ptosis.

QUESTIONS

In surgical exams, ptosis is most likely to be due to Horner's syndrome, possibly secondary to:
- Lower brachial plexus injury (Dejerine–Klumpke paralysis – *see* Case 100)
- Pancoast's tumour of the lung (an apical lung carcinoma that invades the cervical sympathetic plexus, associated with shoulder and arm pain due to brachial plexus invasion of C8–T2, and a hoarse voice or bovine cough due to unilateral recurrent laryngeal nerve palsy and vocal cord paralysis)

(a) What causes of ptosis are you aware of?

Unilateral:

- Third cranial nerve palsy – complete ptosis
- Horner's syndrome – partial ptosis
- Syphilis

Bilateral:

- Congenital ptosis
- Myopathies – myasthenia gravis, dystrophia myotonica
- Syphilis

(b) What surgical treatments are available?

A blepharoplasty can be performed: excess eyelid skin and fat are removed

Henry Pancoast (1875–1939). Professor of Radiology, Pennsylvania, USA.

CASE 20   FACIAL NERVE PALSY   ★ ★

INSTRUCTION

'Have a look at this lady's face.'

APPROACH

In a surgical case, think of surgical causes, e.g. parotid gland tumours, old skull fracture – these result in lower motor neurone palsy of the seventh cranial nerve (facial nerve).

VITAL POINTS

Inspect systematically

- General – loss of facial expression
- Eyelids – on blinking, the affected side closes after the normal eyelid (Bell's sign – the eyeball moves vertically upwards on the abnormal side when the eye is closed)
- Eyes – widened palpebral fissue
- Nasolabial fold – flatter on affected side
- Mouth – the affected side droops and moves less when talking

Test the muscles involved systematically

- Occipitofrontalis – 'raise your eyebrows' – spared in upper motor neurone facial nerve palsy as the forehead has bilateral cortical representation
- Orbicularis oculi – 'close your eyes as tightly as you can'
- Orbicularis oris – 'show me your teeth'
- Buccinator – 'puff out your cheeks'

Look for an obvious cause

- Look for a scar over the parotid gland – indicating iatrogenic facial nerve damage
- Look for parotid gland enlargement
- Look in the external auditory meatus for herpes zoster (Ramsay Hunt syndrome – see below)

Completion

Say that you would like to:

- Take a history to determine the duration and effects of the condition on the patient
- Examine for taste with salt/sweet solutions (involvement of the chorda tympani, an afferent branch of the facial nerve)
- Test the patient's hearing (hyperacusis can result from involvement of the nerve to stapedius muscle, an efferent branch of the facial nerve)

QUESTIONS

(a) What are the causes of facial nerve palsy?

- Intracranial:
  - vascular – cerebrovascular accident
  - tumour – acoustic neuroma
  - infection – meningitis (rarely)
- Intratemporal:
  - infection – acute and chronic otitis media, herpes zoster (Ramsay Hunt syndrome)
  - idiopathic – Bell's palsy (see below)
  - trauma – surgical, accidental, e.g. basal skull fracture
  - tumour – paraganglioma, squamous cell carcinoma of external or middle ear, metastases, e.g. breast
- Extratemporal:
  - tumour – parotid gland malignancy
  - trauma – surgical, accidental, e.g. facial lacerations

ADVANCED QUESTIONS

(a) What are the branches of the facial nerve?

See Fig. 11.

- Motor:
  - nerve to stapedius
  - nerve to posterior belly of digastric
  - five divisions within the parotid gland – temporal, zygomatic, buccal, mandibular and cervical – to supply the muscles of facial expression (such as orbicularis oculi, buccinator and orbicularis oris)
- Secretomotor – via greater superficial petrosal nerve to lacrimal, nasal and palatine glands
- Taste – via chorda tympani to anterior two-thirds of the tongue
- Sensory – uncommon sensory component of facial nerve carrying cutaneous impulses from the anterior wall of the external auditory meatus known as nervus intermedius or pars intermedia of Wrisberg

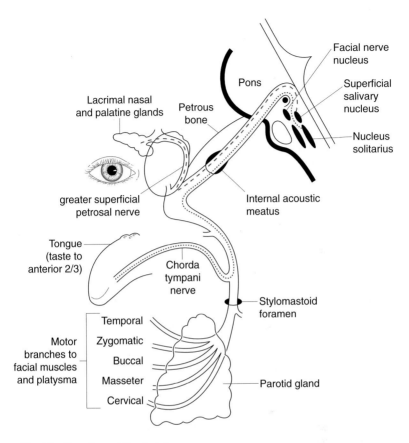

Fig. 11 Branches of the facial nerve.

Sir Charles Bell (1774–1842). Scottish physiologist and Professor of Surgery, Edinburgh who founded the Middlesex Hospital and Medical School, London. He described rapid, unilateral facial weakness associated with or preceded by an ache below the ear which worsens for 1–2 days and then resolves spontaneously within a few days in the majority (85%) of cases. Treatment involves:

- Physiotherapy (massage, electrical stimulation, splint to prevent drooping of the lower part of the face)
- Protection of the eye during sleep, wearing dark glasses during the day and use of artificial tears
- High-dose prednisolone to reduce nerve oedema which prevents weakness becoming paralysis – used if presentation is within a few days of onset

J. Ramsay Hunt (1874–1937). Professor of Neurology, Columbia University, New York. He described involvement of the facial geniculate ganglion with herpes zoster resulting in lower motor neurone facial nerve palsy, severe ear pain and visible vesicles in the external auditory meatus, on the eardrum, on the soft palate or in the tonsillar fossa.

** SALIVARY GLAND SWELLINGS CASE 21

INSTRUCTION

'This gentleman is complaining of a swelling on his right cheek. Examine it and tell me what you think.'

APPROACH

Sit or kneel in front of the patient in order to be at the same level as his face, and examine as for any lump (see Case 1).

VITAL POINTS

Inspect

- Swelling in the region of the parotid gland (which lies wedged between the sternocleidomastoid muscle and the mandible) (Fig. 12) and the submandibular gland (at the angle of the jaw, wedged between the mandible and mylohyoid)
- Look for scars and the opening of a fistula (the latter can occur following parotidectomy or long-standing parotid traumatic injury)
- Stand back and look for facial asymmetry which occurs if the VIIth nerve is involved with a parotid lesion (*see* Case 20)

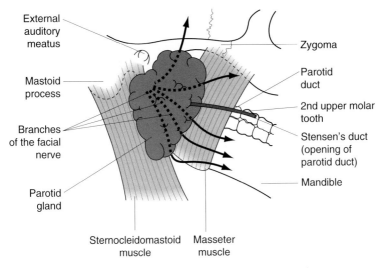

Fig. 12   Anatomy of the right parotid gland.

Palpate from behind

- Walk behind the patient and enquire about tenderness before palpating the swelling
- Is the swelling unilateral or bilateral?
- Is it fixed to the skin or underlying muscle? Ask the patient to clench his teeth, which tenses the masseter and makes the anterior border of the parotid gland more prominent
- Examine for other features as for any lump (*see* Case 1) – see below for features of malignancy
- Continue on to look for cervical lymphadenopathy using the 'up-and-down' routine (*see* Case 6)

Other tests

These tests may be described – in an examination you are unlikely to be asked to perform all of them:

- Look inside the mouth with a pen torch at the opening of the parotid duct (Stensen's duct), which can be found opposite the second upper molar, and at the opening of the submandibular duct (Wharton's duct) on the floor of the mouth adjacent to the frenulum linguae – look for inflammation and pus, or the presence of a stone
- Palpate the parotid duct and submandibular duct openings wearing a pair of gloves, e.g. presence of stone
- Palpate the submandibular gland bimanually with a finger in the mouth and another finger below the angle of the jaw

Finish your examination here

Completion

Say that you would like to:

- Test the facial nerve (*see* Case 20) which may be involved in malignant parotid tumours
- Perform a full ear, nose and throat examination

QUESTIONS

(a) What is the differential diagnosis of a unilateral swelling of the parotid gland?

See Table 12.

Table 12

Arising inside the parotid gland	Arising outside the parotid gland
Neoplasia	Soft-tissues
Benign, e.g. pleomorphic adenoma	Lipoma, sebaceous cyst
Malignant tumours of the parotid	Dental origin
gland	Infection
Lymphoma and leukaemia*	Muscular origin
Stones	Hypertrophy of masseter muscle
Sialolithiasis	Bony origin
Infection/inflammation	Winged mandible
Mumps*	Transverse process of atlas/axis
Acute sialadenitis	Neoplasia
Chronic recurrent sialadenitis	Infratemporal fossa and
Human immunodeficiency virus	parapharyngeal tumours
salivary gland disease	
Autoimmune	
Sjogren's syndrome*	
Infiltration	
Sarcoidosis*	
Lymph node origin	
Parotid lymph node enlargement	
Neural origin	
Facial nerve neuroma	
Vascular origin	
Temporal artery aneurysm	
Systemic diseases	
Alcoholic liver cirrhosis	
Diabetes mellitus	
Pancreatitis	
Acromegaly	
Malnutrition	

*Can present as bilateral swellings

(b) How would you diagnose a benign parotid tumour?

These are adenomas and there are several varieties, the two most important of which are pleomorphic adenoma (most common) and Warthin's tumour (second most common) (Table 13)

Table 13

Pleomorphic adenoma	Warthin's tumour
< 50 years old	> 50 years old
	Smoking important risk factor
Tail of parotid, superficial to upper part of sternomastoid	Tail of parotid, superficial to upper part of sternomastoid
Facial nerve rarely involved	Facial nerve rarely involved

Investigations:

- fine-needle aspiration cytology for diagnosis
- MRI to exclude deep lobe involvement

Surgical treatment is superficial parotidectomy (if superficial lobe of gland only involved) or total parotidectomy with preservation of the facial nerve (if deep lobe of gland or both lobes involved)

(c) What clinical features would make you suspect that a parotid swelling is malignant in nature?

- Rapid growth and pain (on history)
- Hyperaemic hot skin
- Hard consistency
- Fixed to skin and underlying muscle
- Irregular surface or ill-defined edge
- Facial nerve involvement

(d) What is Sjogren's syndrome?

- Autoimmune condition – 90% occur in women at an average age of 50 years
- Intermittent or constant swelling of one or all of the salivary glands
- Clinical diagnosis if at least two of the following triad is present:
  - keratoconjuctivitis sicca (dry eyes)
  - xerostomia (dry mouth)
  - associated connective tissue disorders such as rheumatoid arthritis (50% of cases), scleroderma, systemic lupus erythematosus, polymyositis or polyarteritis nodosa
- If no associated connective tissue disorders are present, this is known as primary Sjogren's disease (note that Mickulicz syndrome is enlargement of the salivary and lacrimal glands secondary to sarcoidosis, lymphoma or tuberculosis, associated with dry mouth and dry eyes, but no arthritis)
- Pathology is lymphocyte-mediated destruction of the exocrine glands secondary to B-cell hyper-reactivity and associated loss of suppressor T-cell activity

- Patients are at $40 \times$ increased risk of developing lymphoma, usually B-cell non-Hodgkin's type
- Several antibodies present, e.g. anti-salivary antibodies, rheumatoid factor, but two specific antibodies present – anti-SSA-Ro and anti-SSB-La
- Other investigations include Schirmer's test for xerophthalmia (strip of filter paper inserted into each fornix and hyposecretion confirmed by wetting of less than 5 mm in 5 minutes – normal is 15 mm), slit-lamp examination of the cornea and lip biopsy for histological examination of the minor salivary glands
- Treatment involves the use of artificial tears and saliva, use of systemic steroids and careful follow-up due to increased risk of lymphoma development

ADVANCED QUESTIONS

(a) What are the complications of parotidectomy?

Specific complications include:

- Immediate
  - facial nerve transection (intraoperative)
  - reactionary haemorrhage
- Early
  - wound infection
  - temporary facial weakness (neuropraxia)
  - salivary fistula
  - division of the greater auricular nerve – loss of sensation to the pinna
- Late
  - Wound dimple
  - Frey's syndrome (auriculotemporal syndrome) – increased sweating of the facial skin when eating, due to reinnervation of divided sympathetic nerves to the facial skin by fibres of the secretomotor branch of the auriculotemporal nerve

---

L. Frey (1889–1944). Polish physician, Warsaw. She was killed by the Nazis.
J. von Mickulicz-Radecki (1850–1905). Professor of Surgery, Breslau, Germany.
O. W. A. Schirmer (1864–1917). German ophthalmologist.
H. S. C. Sjogren (1899–). Professor of Ophthalmology, Gothenburg, Sweden.
N. Stensen (1638–1686). Professor of Anatomy, Copenhagen, Denmark.
A. S. Warthin (1866–1931). Professor of Pathology, Ann Arbor, Michigan, USA.
T. Wharton (1614–1673). English physician, St. Thomas's Hospital, London, UK.

Notes on salivary gland tumours

- 80% of salivary gland tumours occur in the parotid gland, 80% of these parotid tumours being benign, with 80% of these benign tumours being pleomorphic adenomas
- In contrast, only 10% of salivary gland tumours occur in the submandibular gland, with only 60% of these submandibular tumours being benign (i.e. submandibular gland tumours are *twice* as likely to be malignant)
- The only known risk-factor for salivary gland tumours is *exposure to radiation*
- The most common malignant salivary gland tumour is the mucoepidermoid tumour, which is most common in the parotid gland
- The most common malignant salivary gland tumour occurring in the submandibular gland, sublingual gland and the minor salivary glands is adenoid-cystic carcinoma
- The treatment of malignant salivary gland tumours involves total excision of the involved gland with preservation if possible of associated nerves (facial nerve in the case of the parotid gland and the lingual or hypoglossal nerves in the case of the submandibular gland) unless there is direct infiltration of the nerve by tumour. Adjuvant radiotherapy may also be used

CASE 22	KERATOACANTHOMA **

INSTRUCTION

'Examine this gentleman's face.'

APPROACH

Examine as for any lump (*see* Case 1).

VITAL POINTS

- Found on sun-exposed parts of the body
- Commoner in males

Inspect

- Dome-shaped with central crater (containing keratin)
- Normal skin colour (except for the central core which is brown or black due to keratin)

Palpate

- Firm consistency (except for the central core which is hard)
- Fully mobile over deep tissues (as they occur in the skin)

Completion

Say that you would like to ask the patient how the lump affects their lives, e.g. cosmetic symptoms

QUESTIONS

(a) What is a keratoacanthoma?

A keratoacanthoma is a benign overgrowth of hair follicle cells that produces a central plug of keratin. It is rapidly growing, forming within 6 weeks and regressing after 6 weeks, leaving a depressed scar. Clinically and cytologically, they may look similar to well-differentiated squamous cell carcinomas. Occasionally, rapidly growing malignant melanomas may appear similar.

(b) How would you treat this condition?

- Non-surgical – leave alone if asymptomatic (particularly in young patients)
- Surgical – complete excision of lesion with histology (particularly in elderly patients where there should be a high index of suspicion for squamous cell carcinoma)

FURTHER READING

Sullivan J J (1997). Keratoacanthoma: the Australian experience. *Austral J Dermatol* **38** (Suppl 1): S36–9.

** NEUROFIBROMA   CASE 23

INSTRUCTION

No specific instructions – neurofibromata can occur on any part of the body.

APPROACH

Examine as for any lump (Case 1).

VITAL POINTS

Inspect

- May be solitary or multiple (the latter being known as neurofibromatosis – see below)
- Pedunculated nodules
- If arising from deeper nerves, can result in severe deformity due to diffuse enlargement of the peripheral nerve with involvement of the skin (plexiform neurofibroma)

- Look for associated café-au-lait spots in neurofibromatosis (light brown macules which are greater than 1.5 cm in diameter – six or more suggest a diagnosis of neurofibromatosis) – if you see one or two, ask the patient to point out any others he or she may have anywhere else

Palpate

- Soft ('fleshy') in consistency

Completion

Say that you would like to ask the patient:

- How the lump(s) affects their lives, e.g. cosmetic symptoms
- If multiple neurofibromata, say that you would like to test the cranial nerves (particularly the eighth) and measure the blood pressure (associated with phaeochromocytoma)

QUESTIONS

(a) What is a neurofibroma?

A neurofibroma is a benign tumour derived from peripheral nerve elements.

(b) What is neurofibromatosis?

This is the presence of multiple neurofibromas in a patient, in combination with other dermatological manifestations (six café-au-lait spots). It is an autosomal dominant condition. There are thought to be two types of neurofibromatosis:

- Type 1 (Von Recklinghausen's disease) – defective gene on chromosome 17
- Type 2 (bilateral acoustic neurofibromatosis) – defective gene on chromosome 22 with variable penetrance. Cutaneous signs less often seen in this type

(c) What complications can neurofibromata give rise to?

- Pressure effects, e.g. spinal cord and nerve root compression
- Deafness with involvement of the VIIIth cranial nerve
- Sarcomatous transformation – occurs only in Von Recklinghausen's disease in 5–13% of cases
- Intra-abdominal effects – obstruction, chronic gastrointestinal bleeds
- Skeletal changes – can cause kyphoscoliosis, cystic changes and pseudoarthrosis

(d) How would you treat a patient with a single neurofibroma?

- Non-surgical – leave alone if asymptomatic and if patient does not want intervention
- Surgical – indicated only if malignant growth suspected; post-excision, local regrowth is common as neurofibromata cannot be surgically detached from the underlying nerve

ADVANCED QUESTIONS

(a) What is the histological appearance of a neurofibroma?

- Consist of Schwann cells which appear as bundles of elongated wavy spindle cells
- Associated with collagen fibrils and myxoid material
- Often not encapsulated (unlike neurilemmomas – the other common benign tumour of peripheral nerves – which are always encapsulated)

Friedrich Daniel von Recklinghausen (1833–1910). Professor of Pathology, Strasbourg, Germany. Also described von Recklinghausen's Disease of Bone (osteitis fibrosa cystica seen in hyperparathyroidism) and haemochromatosis.

FURTHER READING

Hirsch N P, Murphy A, Radcliffe J J (2001). Neurofibromatosis: clinical presentations and anaesthetic implications. *Br J Anaesth* **86**(4): 555–64.

** PAPILLOMA — CASE 24

INSTRUCTION

No specific instruction.

APPROACH

Examine as for any lump (*see* Case 1).

VITAL POINTS

- Also known as skin tags or fibroepithelial polyps
- Can occur anywhere on the skin, particularly on the neck, trunk, face or anus
- Pedunculated swelling (may be sessile)
- Flesh-coloured
- Soft to palpation

Completion

Say that you would like to ask the patient about:
- Similar lumps elsewhere
- How the lump affects their lives, e.g. cosmetic symptoms
- Associated conditions – there is a link with pregnancy, diabetes and intestinal polyposis

QUESTIONS

(a) What is a papilloma?

A papilloma is an over-growth of all layers of the skin with a central vascular core. They are increasingly common with age.

(b) How would you treat a papilloma?

The simplest surgical technique is to excise the papilloma with a sharp pair of scissors, controlling bleeding from the central vascular component with a single suture. Alternatively, diathermy can be used to control the bleeding at the same time as the excision.

CASE 25   PYOGENIC GRANULOMA   **

INSTRUCTION

'Examine this lady's face.' (Pyogenic granulomata are found most commonly on the hands and face in children and young adults, and on the gums and lips in pregnant women.)

APPROACH

Examine as for any lump (*see* Case 1)

VITAL POINTS

Inspect

- Bright-red or blood encrusted hemispherical nodule
- May be sessile or pedunculated
- May be associated with a serous or purulent discharge
- Can be skin coloured if long standing (epithelialisation)

Palpate

- Soft in consistency ('fleshy')
- Slightly compressible (due to vascular origin)
- May bleed easily (so palpate only if the examiner asks you to)

Completion

Say that you would like to ask the patient:

- Whether they can remember a previous injury in this area (this association with trauma is now thought to be less strong, but show the examiner that you are aware that there is thought to be a link between the two)

- How long the lump took to appear (rapid growth in a few days)
- How the lump affects their lives, e.g. pain, cosmetic symptoms, bleeding

QUESTIONS

(a) What is a pyogenic granuloma?

A pyogenic granuloma is a rapidly growing capillary haemangioma which usually measures less than 1 cm in diameter. It is neither pyogenic nor a granuloma!

(b) How would you treat this condition?

- Non-surgical – regression is uncommon, except those arising in pregnancy, and so they are best treated surgically, though occasionally a silver nitrite stick can be attempted
- Surgical – curettage with diathermy of the base or complete excision biopsy (if recurrent, consider malignancy, e.g. amelanotic melanoma)

** **SEBORRHOEIC KERATOSIS (BASAL CELL PAPILLOMA OR SENILE KERATOSIS)**   **CASE 26**

INSTRUCTION

'Have a look at this lady's face.'

APPROACH

Examine as for any lump (*see* Case 1).

VITAL POINTS

- Commonly found on the trunk and face but can occur anywhere
- Single or multiple
- Round or oval in shape
- 'Stuck-on' appearance
- Varying degree of pigmentation – light brown to black (in black people, seborrhoeic keratoses on the face are known as *dermatosis papulosa nigra)*
- Surface appears velvety or warty
- Can be picked off the skin, leaving behind pink skin and one or two surface capillaries that bleed slightly (*do not attempt to do this in the exam!*)

Completion

Say that you would like to ask the patient:

- About similar lesions elsewhere (note that sudden onset of multiple seborrhoeic keratoses is associated with visceral malignancy – this is known as the Leser–Trelat sign)
- How the lesion affects her life, e.g. cosmetic symptoms, catches on clothes

QUESTIONS

(a) What is a seborrhoeic keratosis?

A seborrhoeic keratosis is a benign overgrowth of the basal cell layer of the epidermis. Histologically, it is characterized by:

- Hyperkeratosis (thickening of the keratin layer)
- Acanthosis (thickening of the prickle cell layer)
- Hyperplasia of variably pigmented basaloid cells

This condition can be confused clinically with acanthosis nigricans.

(b) How would you treat this condition?

- Non-surgical – can be left alone on patient's wishes as it is a benign lesion
- Surgical – as the keratosis lies above the level of the surrounding normal epidermis, it can be treated by superficial shaving or cautery

> E. Leser (1828–1916). German surgeon.
> W. Trelat (1828–1890). French surgeon.

FURTHER READING

Pariser R J (1998) Benign neoplasms of the skin. Med Clin North Am **82**(6): 1285–307.

** SOLAR KERATOSIS (SENILE OR ACTINIC KERATOSIS)   CASE 27

INSTRUCTION

'Have a look at this gentleman's face.' (They are commonly found on sun-exposed parts of the face and dorsum of the hands of elderly people.)

APPROACH

Examine as for any lump (*see* Case 1).

VITAL POINTS

- Usually multiple
- Yellow-grey or brown in colour
- Begin with thickening of skin which can become unsightly and catch on clothing
- Scaly surface
- Can occur as a 'solar horn' on the pinna of the ear – these are also benign

Completion

Say that you would like to ask the patient about:

- Similar lesions elsewhere
- How the lesion affects his life, e.g. cosmetic symptoms

QUESTIONS

(a) What is a solar keratosis?

Solar keratoses are squamous cell carcinomata in situ. Histological appearances include:

- Hyperkeratosis (thickening of the keratin layer)
- Focal parakeratosis
- Irregular acanthosis (thickening of the prickle cell layer)
- Basal layer atypia only (versus atypia in all layers of the epidermis in squamous cell carcinoma – *see* Case 14)

(b) What is the risk of progression to invasive squamous cell carcinoma?

If untreated, 25% progress to invasive squamous cell carcinoma.

(c) How would you treat this condition?

- Non-surgical – cryotherapy, topical application of 5-fluorouracil (cytotoxic agent), retinoic acid (to reverse the damaging effects of sunlight)
- Surgical – shaving of affected skin

FURTHER READING

Dinehart S M (2000) The treatment of actinic keratoses. *J Am Acad Dermatol*
   42(1/2): 25–8.

CASE 28   **DIGITAL CLUBBING**   *

INSTRUCTION

'Examine this patient's hands.'

APPROACH

This case is a spot diagnosis. As for any case involving the hands, expose to above
the elbows and ask the patient to place his hands palm upwards on a pillow (if available). If the instruction is to inspect the nails, then just look at them without going
through this routine.

VITAL POINTS

Inspect

- Exaggerated anteroposterior and longitudinal curvature to fingernails (Fig. 13)
- Loss of angle between nail and nail bed (this can be more clearly seen by
  approximating the dorsal aspects of the terminal phalanges of the fingers of
  both hands after flexing at the interphalangeal joints, and is known as
  Lovibond's sign or the 'diamond sign')
- 'Drumstick' or 'parrot-beak' appearance of the nail (also known as 'doigts
  Hippocratique')

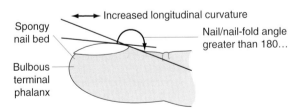

Fig. 13   Digital clubbing.

Palpate

- Increased bogginess/fluctuation of nail bed – elicit this by supporting the
  patient's finger with your two thumbs and use your index fingers to
  demonstrate fluctuance

Completion

Say that you would like to:

- Palpate the wrist joints for tenderness in hypertrophic pulmonary osteoarthropathy (HPOA) – rapid painful digital clubbing is nearly always due to bronchial carcinoma
- Examine the toes to look for digital clubbing
- Take a history and examine the patient to elicit the duration of digital clubbing, e.g. is it from birth, and to look for underlying causes (see below)

TOP TIP

Note that the correct term is 'digital clubbing' – the word clubbing on its own may have several connotations, e.g. something done on a Friday night!

QUESTIONS

(a) What are the causes of digital clubbing?

The most common cause of clubbing is *idiopathic*. The other causes can be divided into:

- Gastrointestinal:
  - liver cirrhosis (especially primary biliary cirrhosis)
  - inflammatory bowel disease (especially Crohn's disease)
  - malabsorption (coeliac disease, tropical sprue)
  - gastrointestinal lymphoma
- Respiratory:
  - bronchial carcinoma (most commonly squamous cell)
  - chronic suppurative lung disease (abscess, bronchiectasis, cystic fibrosis, empyema)
  - fibrosing alveolitis
  - mesothelioma
- Cardiac:
  - cyanotic congenital heart diseases (e.g. Fallot's tetralogy, transposition of the great arteries)
  - infective endocarditis
  - atrial myxoma (rare)
- Rare causes:
  - familial, e.g. 'hazel nails' (usually seen before puberty), pachydermoperiostitis (idiopathic familial HPOA with postpubertal digital clubbing, bone changes, increased sweating of palms and soles and marked thickening of the skin, forehead and scalp)
  - Grave's disease (pseudoclubbing – also known as thyroid acropachy)
  - unilaterally seen in axillary artery aneurysm and brachial arteriovenous malformation

ADVANCED QUESTIONS

(a) What do you know about the pathophysiology of digital clubbing?

Several theories have been put forward to try and explain the mechanisms behind digital clubbing. They include:

- Vasodilatation of nail-bed vessels secondary to an unidentified mediator (candidates include ferritin, bradykinin, prostaglandin and 5-hydroxytryptamine), which is normally inactivated in the lung but may persist in those with digital clubbing where inactivation is defective or there is a right-to-left shunt
- Increased growth hormone
- Organs supplied by the vagus are affected by digital clubbing – vagotomy can reverse digital clubbing in bronchial carcinoma
- Tumour necrosis factor
- Increased platelet-derived growth factor and fibroblast growth factor resulting in increased fibroblastic activity, capillary permeability and arterial smooth muscle hyperplasia

(b) How do you grade digital clubbing?

- Grade I: increased glossiness and cyanosis of the skin at the root of the nail associated with increased fluctuation at the base of the nail bed
- Grade II: loss of angle between nail and nail bed (see above)
- Grade III: drumstick appearance of nail (see above)
- Grade IV: bony changes involving the wrists and ankles, sometimes the elbow and knees (HPOA)

Hippocrates (460–379 BC). Greek physician, born in Kos, commonly thought of as the founder of medicine.

E. L. A. Fallot (1850–1911). Professor of Hygiene and Legal Medicine, Marseilles, France. He described congenital cyanotic heart disease due to a combination of 1. ventricular septal defect, 2. right ventricular outflow tract obstruction, 3. right ventricular hypertrophy and 4. overriding aorta.

FURTHER READING

Myers KA and Farquhar DR (2001). Does this patient have clubbing? *JAMA* **286**(3): 341–7.
Martinez-Lavin M (1997) Hypertrophic osteoarthropathy *Curr Opin Rheumatol* **9**(1): 83–6.

Notes

Hippocrates first described digital clubbing over 2400 years ago.

| *   **BRANCHIAL CYST** | **CASE 29** |

INSTRUCTION

'Examine this gentleman's neck.'

APPROACH

Approach as for neck examination (*see* Case 6).

VITAL POINTS

- Usually presents in a young adult in the third decade
- Equally common in males and females
- Found in anterior triangle of neck in front of the upper or middle third of the sternocleidomastoid
- Smooth, firm swelling that is ovoid in shape with its long axis running forwards and downwards
- Fluctuant on palpation
- Usually opaque on transillumination (due to desquamated epithelial cell contents)
- May be hard and fixed to surrounding structures in the presence of established or recurrent infection
- Look carefully for the opening of a fistula in this area (a branchial fistula runs between the tonsillar fossa and the anterior border of the sternocleidomastoid)

TOP TIP

There are three surgical definitions that you should be able to roll off your tongue:

- Cyst – an abnormal sac containing gas, fluid or semisolid material, with an epithelial lining
- Sinus – a blind-ending track, typically lined by epithelial or granulation tissue, which opens onto an epithelial surface
- Fistula – an abnormal communication between two epithelial surfaces (*or endothelial surfaces*, e.g. arteriovenous fistula)

Completion

Say that you would like to ask the patient about:

- Associated symptoms, e.g. pain, symptoms of infection
- The effect of the lump on his life

QUESTIONS

(a) What is a branchial cyst?

A branchial cyst is thought to develop because of a failure of fusion of the embryonic second and third branchial arches. An alternative, and currently popular, hypothesis is that it is an acquired condition due to cystic degeneration in cervical lymphatic tissue. The cysts are lined by squamous epithelium.

(b) How would you diagnose a branchial cyst?

- Clinical examination
- Fine-needle aspiration – opalescent fluid containing cholesterol crystals or pus

(c) How would you treat a branchial cyst?

- The cyst may be surgically excised – whole if possible, although this may be difficult if there has been previous infection
- Bonney's blue dye can be injected into the fistula/sinus allowing accurate surgical excision and therefore reduces recurrence rates
- Complicating infections may be treated with antibiotics
- Complications include recurrence of the cyst and development of a chronic, discharging sinus

FURTHER READING

Davenport M (1996) ABC of general surgery in children. Lumps and swellings of the head and neck. *BMJ* **312**(7027): 368–71.

http://www.pedisurg.com/PtEduc/Branchial_Cleft_Cyst.htm – information for parents on their children's neck lumps.

CASE 30   DERMOID CYST   *

INSTRUCTION

No specific instruction – can occur in various sites.

APPROACH

Examine as for any lump (*see* Case 1).

VITAL POINTS

Inspect

- Smooth spherical swelling
- Soft and may fluctuate

- Non-tender
- Look for associated scar from previous injury (especially in adults)

> **TOP TIP**
> Dermoid cysts lie deep to the skin in the subcutaneous tissues. They differ from lipomas as they are not within the fat layers, and from sebaceous cysts as they are not attached to skin.

Completion

Say that you would like to ask the patient:

- How the cyst affects their lives, e.g. cosmetic symptoms
- Whether they have suffered an injury previously (if you suspect that it is an acquired cyst)

QUESTIONS

(a) What is a dermoid cyst?

- A dermoid cyst is a skin-lined cyst deep to the skin. They may be congenital or acquired
- Congenital – due to developmental inclusion of epidermis along lines of fusion of skin dermatomes and are therefore found commonly at:
  - the medial and lateral ends of the eyebrows (internal and external angular dermoid cysts)
  - the midline of the nose (nasal dermoid cysts)
  - the midline of the neck and trunk

  Suspect if you see a *child* or *young adult* in the exam
- Acquired – due to forced implantation of skin into subcutaneous tissues following an injury. Normally found in areas of the body prone to injury such as fingers. Suspect if you see an *adult* in exam

(b) How would you treat this condition?

- Congenital – surgical treatment involves complete excision but the full extent of the cyst should be established with suitable radiographic views (X-ray or CT scan)
- This is especially important in midline cysts which may communicate with the cerebrospinal fluid so exclusion of a bony defect is vital before surgery
- Acquired – surgical treatment involves complete excision of the cyst

FURTHER READING

Rosen D, Wirtschafter A, Rao V M, Wilcox T O Jr (1998) Dermoid cyst of the lateral neck: a case report and literature review. *Ear Nose Throat J* **77**(2): 129–32.

CASE 31	THYROGLOSSAL CYST *

INSTRUCTIONS

'Examine this gentleman's neck.'

APPROACH

Approach as you would a neck examination (*see* Case 6).

Inspect (FROM THE FRONT)

- Site of the lump – note that 75% are in the midline, 25% are either a little to the right or the left
- Smooth and rounded
- Other features on inspection of the lump, e.g. size, skin changes (you may see the opening of a thyroglossal sinus with seropurulent discharge, which follows rupture or incision of a thyroglossal cyst), scars (*see* Case 8)

Protrusion of the tongue

- Ask the patient to open his mouth and stick his tongue out as far as possible
- If the lump moves on protrusion of the tongue, it is likely to be a thyroglossal cyst (this is because the cyst is usually related to the base of the tongue by a patent or fibrous track which runs through the central portion of the hyoid bone) – a lump from the thyroid gland does not move on protrusion of the tongue

Swallowing

- Place a glass of water in the patient's hands, ask him to take a sip of water, hold it in his mouth and swallow when you ask him to
- As he swallows, inspect the lump – if it moves on swallowing, it is likely to originate from the thyroid gland
- Note that thyroglossal cysts also move on swallowing, so ask the patient to stick his tongue out before proceeding with the thyroid gland examination (*see* Case 8)

Palpate (FROM THE BACK)

Repeat the two above tests, this time palpating the cyst gently from behind the patient to ensure that the diagnosis is correct

Finish your examination here

Completion

Say that you would like to:

- Take a history from the patient, particularly concentrating on how the lump affects his life, e.g. cosmetic symptoms

QUESTIONS

(a) What is your differential diagnosis?

The differential diagnosis includes other midline neck lumps:

- Thyroid nodules and masses (including pyramidal lobe)
- Enlarged lymph nodes
- Other cysts – dermoid and epidermoid
- Subhyoid bursae

(b) What do you know about the epidemiology of thyroglossal cysts?

- Rare
- Worldwide distribution
- Equally common in males and females
- Rarely present at birth, 40% present in the first decade and can even present late in the ninth decade

(c) How do you treat a thyroglossal cyst?

- Treatment is essentially surgical
- Operation of choice is Sistrunk's operation
- Inject patent track with dye at the start of the operation
- Excise cyst and the patent or fibrous track which runs through the central portion of the hyoid bone (which is also excised)
- May have to dissect up to the origin at the foramen caecum (see below)
- If central portion of hyoid bone not excised, high incidence of recurrence

ADVANCED QUESTIONS

(a) What is the embryological origin of a thyroglossal cyst?

- Results from persistence of part of the thyroglossal tract, which marks the developmental descent of the thyroid gland
- At the fourth week of development, the thyroid appears as a midline diverticulum and descends ventrally to the pharynx between the developing second arch as a duct (which normally involutes)
- The origin of the tract can persist as a midline dimple – the foramen caecum – at the junction of the valate and filiform papillae of the tongue

(b) What are the pathological features of thyroglossal cysts?

- Lined by stratified squamous or ciliated pseudostratified columnar epithelium
- May also contain thyroid or lymphoid tissue, which can undergo malignant change
- If malignancy occurs, usually of thyroid papillary type

FURTHER READING

Brewis C, Mahadevan M, Bailey C M, Drake D P (2000) Investigation and treatment of thyroglossal cysts in children. *J R Soc Med* **93**(1): 18–21.

CASE 32	RADIOTHERAPY MARKS *

INSTRUCTION

'Have a look at this lady's chest.'

APPROACH

As this is a spot diagnosis, the patient should be adequately exposed to their waist – if they are covered up, explain what you are going to do and obtain sufficient exposure. Approach as you would a breast examination (*see* Case 63).

VITAL POINTS

Inspect

- For any evidence of chest wall or breast disease – the patient may have undergone a unilateral mastectomy

Current radiotherapy

- India-ink marks
- Erythema
- Desquamation
- Skin markings to delineate area of treatment

Previous radiotherapy

- Telangectasia

Completion

Say that you would like to:

- Take a history to determine the duration and side-effects of radiotherapy on this lady

ADVANCED QUESTIONS

(a) How does radiotherapy work?

High-energy X-rays interact with tissues to release electrons of high kinetic energy, which cause secondary damage to adjacent DNA via an oxygen-dependent mechanism. The damage is either repairable or non-repairable, the latter manifesting itself as chromosomal abnormalities preventing mitosis. Normal tissues have a greater ability to repopulate in response to radiation-induced cell depletion than do tumours.

(b) Which normal tissues are particularly affected by radiotherapy?

Tissues with rapid turnover:

- Epidermal layers of the skin
- Small intestine
- Bone marrow stem cells

Tissues with a limited ability to repopulate:

- Spinal cord
- Gonads – oocytes and spermatocytes

(c) What are the side-effects of radiotherapy?

Early:

- General – malaise, fatigue, loss of appetite, nausea and vomiting
- Skin – as above
- Bone marrow suppression – particularly if irradiation to the pelvis and long bones
- Gastrointestinal – diarrhoea

Late:

- Skin – as above
- Lungs – pneumonitis, pulmonary fibrosis
- Heart – ischaemic heart disease
- Arteries – radiation arteritis, especially the carotids post head and neck radiotherapy; this leads to subsequent stenosis and distal ischaemia
- Spinal cord – myelopathy
- Visceral damage – constricted fibrotic bladder, bowel obstruction secondary to strictures and adhesions, renal impairment due to depletion of renal tubular cells
- Gonadal damage – infertility
- Thyroid – hypothyroidism due to depletion of thyroid follicular cells
- Eyes – cataracts
- Secondary malignancies – increased risk of solid tumours and also of leukaemias (the risk of the latter being 1–2% at 15 years, with an even higher risk if chemotherapy with alkylating agents are used in conjunction)

(d) How are the side-effects of radiotherapy minimized?

- Lead shields to protect the eyes and gonads
- Dose fractionation – to allow recovery of normal host tissues
- Prior chemotherapy – to increase sensitivity of tumour to radiotherapy
- Regional hypothermia – useful in superficial tumours and bulky non-vascular tumours
- Radiolabelled antibodies – delivering high levels of radiation locally to the tumour

CASE 33   DERMATOFIBROMA   *

INSTRUCTION

'Examine this lady's legs.'

APPROACH

Examine as for any lump (*see* Case 1).

VITAL POINTS

Inspect

- Can occur anywhere but are more common on the lower limbs of young to middle-aged women
- Small pink or brown pigmented hemispherical nodules
- Smooth in appearance

Palpate

- Firm woody feel (characteristic)
- They are part of the skin and are therefore fully mobile over deep tissues

Completion

Say that you would like to ask the patient:

- What symptoms they are experiencing from the lump, e.g. cosmetic

QUESTIONS

(a) What is a dermatofibroma?

A dermatofibroma (also known as a fibrous histiocytoma) is a benign neoplasm of dermal fibroblasts. Previous theories that dermatofibromas are a reaction to a previous injury or insect bite have now fallen out of favour. Recent thinking favours the concept that it is a result of an abortive immunoreactive process, featuring dermal dendritic cells as initiators of the disease.

(b) What is the differential diagnosis?

It is important to exclude malignant tumours such as:

- Malignant melanoma (*see* Case 15)
- Basal cell carcinoma (*see* Case 16)

(c) How would you treat this condition?

- Non-surgical – leave alone if asymptomatic and if patient does not want intervention
- Surgical – simple excision followed by histology

FURTHER READING

Nestle F O, Nickoloff B J, Burg G (1995) Dermatofibroma: an abortive immunoreactive process mediated by dermal dendritic cells? *Dermatology* **190**(4): 265–8.

http://www.skinsite.com/info_dermatofibromas.htm – information for patients.

---

* HIDRADENITIS SUPPURATIVA CASE 34

INSTRUCTION

'Examine this lady's left axilla.'

APPROACH

Examine as for any lump (*see* Case 1).

VITAL POINTS

- The skin is thickened and may be ulcerated; 'watering-can' sinuses may be seen
- Look for signs of any active current infection (tenderness/increased temperature/erythema)

COMPLETION

Say that you would like to ask the patient about:

- Symptoms arising from this condition and how they affect the patient
- Any other affected areas, e.g. perineum, groins
- Predisposing factors, e.g. diabetes mellitus

QUESTIONS

(a) What is hidradenitis suppurativa?

Hidradenitis suppurativa is a chronic and recurrent infection of the apocrine sweat glands. It is thought to be due to an antigen–antibody reaction with blockage of follicular secretions and subsequent abscess formation. Other theories are based on the concept that it is due to a defect of terminal follicular epithelium. Abscesses form recurrently and this causes the characteristic permanent disfiguring of the skin. It usually affects young women, with a prevalence of 0.3–0.4% in industrialized countries.

(b) How would you treat hidradenitis suppurativa?

Hidradenitis can be extremely uncomfortable, cosmetically unpleasant and distressing for the patient; they are also problematic to treat satisfactorily.

- Well-localized abscess – incision and drainage under antibiotic cover
- Larger lesions – radical excision and full-thickness skin grafting usually harvested from the groins or abdomen

FURTHER READING

Brown T J, Rosen T, Orengo I F (1998). Hidradenitis suppurativa. *South Med J* **91**(12): 1107–14.

CASE 35   KAPOSI'S SARCOMA   *

INSTRUCTION

'Have a look at this skin lesion.'

APPROACH

Examine as for any lump (*see* Case 1).

VITAL POINTS

Inspect

- Purple papules or plaques
- Solitary or multiple
- Can be found anywhere on skin or on mucosa of any organ but usually found on the limbs, mouth, tip of the nose or palate

Completion

Say that you would like to:
- Take a history, e.g. ethnic origin, previous transplant
- Ask the patient about underlying immunocompromise (without saying 'HIV' or 'AIDS' directly)

QUESTIONS

(a) What do you know about Kaposi's sarcoma?

- Derived from capillary endothelial cells or from fibrous tissue
- Linked to human herpes virus 8 (HHV-8) – also known as Kaposi's sarcoma herpes virus (KSHV)

(b) How would you treat this condition?

- Leave alone if asymptomatic and if patient does not want intervention
- Intervene only when extensive or for cosmetic reasons:
  - local radiotherapy
  - chemotherapy – interferon-α, doxorubicin, intralesional vinblastine

Mention that Kaposi's is usually present in advanced HIV infection and so adequate anti-retroviral therapy is required.

ADVANCED QUESTIONS

(a) What varieties do you know of Kaposi's sarcoma?

- Classic Kaposi's sarcoma:
  - initially described in Ashkenazi Jews
  - found on the legs of elderly men
  - confined to skin
  - not fatal
- AIDS-associated Kaposi's sarcoma
  - found in one-third of patients with AIDS (diagnostic of AIDS)
  - more common in homosexual patients
  - one-third develop a second malignancy, e.g. leukaemia, lymphoma
- Endemic (central African) variety
  - aggressive invasive tumour
  - ultimately fatal
  - good response to chemotherapy
- Transplantation-associated Kaposi's sarcoma
  - following high-dose immunosuppressive therapy
  - often regress when treatment stopped

Moricz Kaposi (1837–1902). Hungarian dermatologist. Also described the rash in systemic lupus erythematosus as a 'butterfly rash' and xeroderma pigmentosum (Kaposi's disease).

FURTHER READING

Aboulafia D M (2001) Kaposi's sarcoma. *Clin Dermatol* **19**(3): 269–83.

Sturzl M, Zietz C, Monini P, and Ensoli B (2001) Human herpesvirus-8 and Kaposi's sarcoma: relationship with the multistep concept of tumorigenesis. *Adv Cancer Res* **81**: 125–59.

CASE 36   PHARYNGEAL POUCH   *

INSTRUCTION

'Examine this gentleman's neck.'

APPROACH

Approach as for neck examination (*see* Case 14).

VITAL POINTS

- Most commonly seen in the elderly
- May be very little to find except for a cystic swelling low down in the anterior triangle of the neck (Fig. 14)
- Deep palpation produces a squelching sound due to free fluid in the pouch
- Halitosis is a frequent feature, as food is regurgitated into the neck

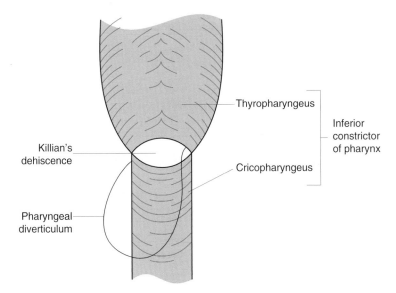

Killian's dehiscence

Thyropharyngeus

Inferior constrictor of pharynx

Cricopharyngeus

Pharyngeal diverticulum

Fig. 14 Anatomy of the pharyngeal pouch.

Completion

Say that you would like to ask the patient about:

- Associated symptoms, e.g. regurgitation leading to coughing, dysphagia
- Complications (see below)
- The effect of the lump on his life

Ask to listen to the patient's chest.

QUESTIONS

(a) What is a pharyngeal pouch?

A pharyngeal pouch is formed by the herniation of pharyngeal mucosa (known as a pulsion diverticulum) through its muscular coat at its weakest point (Killian's dehiscence) between the thyropharyngeal and cricopharyngeal muscles that make up the inferior constrictor. Patients are usually symptom-free for a long period of time followed by dysphagia and hoarseness, associated with regurgitation of un-digested foods, and associated weight-loss.

(b) What are the complications of a pharyngeal pouch?

- Chest infection – due to pulmonary aspiration
- Diverticular neoplasia – in less than 1% of cases

(c) What investigations would you perform to help you in your diagnosis?

- Barium swallow – usually diagnostic
- Rigid endoscopy – if neoplasia suspected

(d) How would you treat a pharyngeal pouch?

- Non-surgical:
  – Leave alone if small and asymptomatic
- Surgical:
  – Minimally invasive surgery – Dohlman's procedure – endoscopic diathermy resection of the posterior pharyngeal wall (used in patients medically unfit for surgical excision), or endoscopic stapling – less risk of fistula formation and consequent mediastinitis
  – Surgical excision – simple inversion and oversewing (diverticulopexy) – as pouch is left *in situ*, risk of missing a possible diverticular carcinoma, or diverticulectomy

FURTHER READING

Siddiq M A, Sood S, Strachan D (2001) Pharyngeal pouch (Zenker's diverticulum). *Postgrad Med J* **77**(910): 506–11.

CASE 37   **CYSTIC HYGROMA**   *

INSTRUCTION

'Examine this gentleman's neck.'

APPROACH

Approach as for neck examination (*see* Case 6) – note these patients are more frequently found in paediatric cases.

VITAL POINTS

- 50–65% are present at birth, but occasionally may present late in late childhood or adulthood
- Located in the posterior triangle of the neck
- Lobulated cystic swelling
- Soft and fluctuant
- Compressible (usually into another part of the cyst)
- 'Brilliantly transilluminable'

Completion

Say that you would like to:

- Look in the oropharynx (a large cyst may extend deeply beneath the sternocleidomastoid muscle into the retropharyngeal space)
- Ask the patient how the lump affects his life

QUESTIONS

(a) What is a cystic hygroma?

A cystic hygroma is a congenital cystic lymphatic malformation found in the posterior triangle of the neck. It is probably a developmental anomaly formed during the coalescence of primitive lymph elements. It consists of thin-walled, single or multiple interconnecting or separate cysts which insinuate themselves widely into the tissues at the root of the neck.

(b) What are the complications of a cystic hygroma?

Complications include cosmetic symptoms but important problems are encountered in the perinatal period:

- Before delivery:
  - may obstruct delivery
- After delivery
  - respiratory obstruction
  - obstruction of swallowing

(c) What investigations would you perform to help you in your diagnosis?

Investigations are mainly radiological:

- Chest X-ray – to map the caudal extent of the cystic hygroma
- CT/MRI scanning – especially if complex

(d) How would you treat a cystic hygroma?

- Non-surgical:
  – aspiration and injection of sclerosant (generally unsuccessful)
- Surgical:
  – excision – may be partial (to relieve symptoms) or complete (as a one-stage procedure)

FURTHER READING

Fonkalsrud E W (1994) Congenital malformations of the lymphatic system. Review. *Semin Pediatr Surg* **3**(2): 62–9.

Gallagher P G, Mahoney M J, Gosche J R (1999) Cystic hygroma in the fetus and newborn. *Semin Perinatol* **23**(4): 341–56.

http://www.cystichygroma.co.uk/ – support group and networking forum for children and parents affected by lymphatic malformations.

* CHEMODECTOMA CASE 38

INSTRUCTION

'Examine this gentleman's neck.'

APPROACH

Approach as for neck examination (*see* Case 6).

VITAL POINTS

- Located in the anterior triangle of the neck, at the angle of the jaw
- Be gentle when examining in this area as pressure on the carotid bifurcation can induce a vasovagal attack
- Usually the lump is solid and firm
- Pulsatile but not expansile in nature – (be extra gentle as soon as you realise it is pulsatile!) – may be due to:
  – transmitted pulsation from the adjacent carotid arteries
  – an overlying palpable external carotid artery
  – true expansile pulsation from a soft or very vascular tumour

- Due to intimate relationship with the carotid arteries, the lump can be moved from side to side but not up and down
- May be bilateral

QUESTIONS

(a) What is a chemodectoma?

A chemodectoma is a tumour of the paraganglion cells of the carotid body located at the bifurcation of the common carotid artery. They are usually benign (but locally invasive), but occasionally, they are malignant with potential to metastasize to local lymph nodes.

(b) What investigations would you perform to help you in your diagnosis?

- Doppler ultrasound
- Angiography – gold standard – shows a hypervascular mass displacing the bifurcation of the carotid arteries
- CT/MRI – to delineate the extent of the tumour

(d) How would you treat a chemodectoma?

- Surgical:
  - surgical excision (with preoperative embolization if the tumour is large)
  - ultrasonic surgical dissection may also be used
- Radiotherapy:
  - for patients unfit for surgery
  - for large tumours

FURTHER READING

Wang S J, Wang M B, Barauskas T M, Calcaterra T C (2000) Surgical management of carotid body tumors. *Otolaryngol Head Neck Surg* **123**(3): 202–6.

CASE 39   FURUNCLES   *

INSTRUCTION

'Examine this gentleman's right axilla.'

APPROACH

Examine as for any lump (*see* Case 1). These are common in Accident and Emergency but are rare in examinations.

VITAL POINTS

- Can affect any hair-bearing area of the skin, particularly the face, neck, buttocks, groins and axillae
- Small pus-containing swelling (when the contents become solid, it is known as a boil)
- Tender on palpation
- May be multiple

Completion

Say that you would like to ask the patient about:

- Other affected areas
- Predisposing factors such as diabetes mellitus, steroid treatment and other immunodeficiencies

Ask to test the urine or blood for sugar.

QUESTIONS

(a) What is a furuncle?

A furuncle results from infection of hair follicles with *Staphylococcus aureus*.

(b) How would you treat this condition?

- Non-surgical – risk-factor modification, e.g. establishment of good diabetic control and, for recurrent infections, eradication of nasal carriage of *Staphylococcus aureus* with antiseptics and/or antibiotics, e.g. chlorhexidine and mupirocin
- Surgical – incision and drainage for large and painful boils

(c) What is a carbuncle?

A carbuncle is an extensive infection of hair follicles by the same organism, with involvement of adjacent follicles and development of draining sinuses. It is associated with diabetes and is treated with a combination of systemic antibiotics and surgical incision.

FURTHER READING

Williams R E, MacKie R M (1993) The staphylococci. Importance of their control in the management of skin disease. *Dermatol Clin* **11**(1): 201–6

CASE 40 — PYODERMA GANGRENOSUM *

INSTRUCTION

No specific instruction – lesion can be on any part of the body but usually found on the trunk, lower limbs or face

APPROACH

Examine as for ulcers (*see* Case 1)

VITAL POINTS

Inspect

- Ulcer with necrotic base
- Irregular bluish-red overhanging edges
- Associated with surrounding erythematous plaques with pustules

Completion

Say that you would like to take a history and examine the patient for evidence of:

- Ulcerative colitis (the presence of pyoderma gangrenosum is related to disease activity)
- Crohn's disease
- Rheumatoid arthritis

QUESTIONS

This is likely to continue on to questions concerning inflammatory bowel disease, particularly ulcerative colitis (Case 50)

ADVANCED QUESTIONS

(a) What other associations of pyoderma gangrenosum do you know of?

- Idiopathic (50%)
- Myleoproliferative disorders, e.g. polycythaemia rubra vera, myeloma
- Autoimmune hepatitis
- More common in males than females

(b) What is your differential diagnosis?

- Autoimmune:
  – rheumatoid vasculitis

- Infectious:
  - tertiary syphilis
  - amoebiasis
- Iatrogenic:
  - Warfarin necrosis
- Unknown:
  - Behcet's disease

(c) How would you treat this condition?

- Medical – treat underlying condition, saline cleansing, high-dose oral or intralesional steroids +/– cyclosporin +/– antibiotics
- Surgical – serial allograft followed by autologous skin graft or muscle flap coverage when necessary

---

Hulusi Behcet (1889–1948). Professor to the Clinic of Dermatology and Syphilis, Turkey. Multi-organ disease of unknown (viral?) aetiology causing arthritis, pyoderma, ulcers in the mouth, scrotum and labia, eye problems such as hypopyon (pus in the anterior chamber of the eye) and iritis, and with central nervous involvement, e.g. meningoencephalitis. Most common geographically along the Silk Road and is linked with HLA-B51.

FURTHER READING

Rozen S M, Nahabedian M Y, Manson P N (2001) Management strategies for pyoderma gangrenosum: case studies and review of literature. *Ann Plast Surg* **47**(3): 310–5.

---

* **VASCULAR MALFORMATIONS**   **CASE 41**

GENERAL

These are unlikely cases but a few points are described below in case they are pointed out during the course of your examinations. Some of these conditions may occur in paediatrics short cases or OSCEs.

TYPES

- Capillary – account for two-thirds of all cases and include naevi, port-wine stains, telangectasiae and spider naevi
- Predominantly venous – venous angioma
- Predominantly lymphatic – lymphangioma circumscriptum (*see* Case 130)

COMMON FEATURES

- Develop as an abnormal proliferation of the embryonic vascular network
- Hamartomas
- May ulcerate
- May induce hyperkeratosis in the overlying stratum corneum layer of the skin

SPECIFIC LESIONS

Campbell de Morgan's spots

- Small red capillary naevus
- Develops on the trunk in middle-age
- No clinical significance

Spider naevus (also known as naevus araneus)

- Form of telengectasis
- Central arteriole with leg-like branches which blanch on central pressure
- Found over upper torso, head and neck in adults (thought to be within the drainage area of the superior vena cava)
- Associated with chronic liver disease and pregnancy
- More than five is considered as pathological in chronic liver disease

Telangectasis

- Dilatation of normal capillaries
- Can be secondary to skin irradiation (*see* Case 32)
- Can be part of hereditary haemorrhagic telangiectasia (Osler–Rendu–Weber syndrome) – rare autosomal dominant disease (with incomplete penetrance) in which overt and occult haemorrhage can occur presenting as haematuria, haemetemesis, malaena, epistaxis or iron-deficiency anaemia

Port-wine stain (also known as naevus vinosus)

- Purple-blue naevus found on face, lips and mucous membranes of the mouth
- Present from birth and does not change in size thereafter
- Found on limbs in association with Klippel–Trenaunay syndrome (*see* Case 109)
- Sturge–Weber syndrome is the association of a facial port-wine stain with a corresponding haemangioma in the brain, leading to contralateral focal fits

Strawberry patch (cavernous haemangioma)

- Bright-red raised strawberry-like lesion
- Present from birth, but 60% undergo spontaneous resolution by the age of 3
- Only treated if obscuring a visual field or spontaneous resolution not occurring

Campbell de Morgan (1811–1876). Full Surgeon to the Middlesex Hospital in London, who believed the spots were a sign of cancer.

Sir William Osler (1849–1919). Canadian-born Professor of Medicine at McGill, Pennsylvania, Johns Hopkins and Oxford. Also described Osler's nodes (cutaneous nodules in infective endocarditis) and Osler-Vaquez disease (polycythaemia rubra vera).

Henry Jules Louis Marie Rendu (1844–1902). Parisian Physician at the Necker Hospital.

William Allen Sturge (1850–1919). English Physician and Pathologist at the Royal Free Hospital.

Frederick Parkes Weber (1863–1962). English Physician.

ABDOMEN AND TRUNK

CASE 42   INGUINAL HERNIA   ★★★

INSTRUCTION

'Examine this gentleman's groin.'

APPROACH

Expose the patient from umbilicus to knees.

VITAL POINTS

> TOP TIP 1
> Should the hernia be examined with the patient lying down or standing up?
> The answer is that it doesn't matter. It is generally considered to be easier to
> define the anatomy with the patient supine, and if the hernia can be detected
> with the patient on the couch, then examine them there. If no lump can be
> felt, or if no couch is available, then stand the patient up first

> TOP TIP 2
> Don't forget that the same opening instruction may apply to the examination
> of the scrotum, and it may be a scrotal lump rather than a hernia and if you
> cannot see a visible swelling proceed by asking the patient where the lump is

Inspect

- Look at the groin for old surgical scars (is the hernia recurrent?)
- If the hernia is obvious, then begin to examine it.
- If it cannot be seen then ask the patient where the lump is: 'Have you noticed a lump in your groin sir?'

Palpate

- Begin by defining the anatomy
- Palpate the pubic tubercle and the anterior superior iliac spine, demonstrating that the inguinal ligament runs between the two (Fig. 15)
- Show that the hernia arises above this line
- Demonstrate that the lump has an expansile cough impulse: place one hand over the lump and ask the patient to cough
- Other aspects of the lump (as for any lump) may be defined at this stage, e.g. skin changes
- Decide whether the lump is confined to the inguinal region or descends into the scrotum

- Ask the patient if they can ever reduce the hernia: 'Does the lump ever go back inside – can you push it back in for me?'
- If they can push the hernia back, try to control the hernia at the deep inguinal ring. Redefine the inguinal ligament again. When the patient has pushed the hernia back, place two fingers halfway along the inguinal ligament. Ask the patient to cough. If the hernia is controlled by your fingers at the deep inguinal ring it is an INDIRECT inguinal hernia. Remember that the accuracy of clinical examination in distinguishing a direct from an indirect hernia is low (e.g. 56% of direct herniae were wrongly classified by consultant surgeons as indirect on clinical examination in one such study – see further reading)

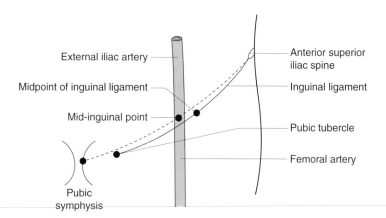

Fig. 15 Anatomy of the inguinal ligament

TOP TIP 3

The pubic tubercle can be difficult to palpate but forms the point of insertion of the prominent adductor longus tendon, running medially up the thigh (the tendon can be made more prominent by flexing, abducting and externally rotating the patient's thigh)

Completion

Complete your examination by asking to examine the scrotum for incidental scrotal lumps and to examine the contralateral groin for herniae.

QUESTIONS

(a) What is the difference between a direct and an indirect inguinal hernia?

Indirect inguinal herniae:

- Are the remnants of a patent processus vaginalis
- Arise from the abdominal cavity, passing obliquely through the deep inguinal ring and travelling through the inguinal canal with the spermatic cord
- May continue through the superficial inguinal ring into the scrotum

Direct inguinal herniae:

- Are the result of a weak posterior wall to the inguinal canal
- This weakness causes the abdominal contents to bulge through the wall into the inguinal canal but the hernia is not within the spermatic cord

(b) What are the contents of the spermatic cord?

Three arteries:
- Artery to vas deferens (from inferior vesicular artery)
- Testicular artery (from aorta)
- Cremasteric artery (from inferior epigastric artery)

Three nerves:
- Ilioinguinal nerve (L1) on the front of the cord
- Nerve to cremaster (from genitofemoral nerve)
- Autonomic nerves (sympathetic fibres from T10)

Three other structures:
- Vas deferens
- Pampiniform plexus of veins (drains right testis into inferior vena cava and left testis into renal vein)
- Lymphatics (drain the testis to the para-aortic lymph nodes)

(c) What would you tell patients about their recovery from inguinal hernia repair?

- Early mobilization from 10 days is important
- They should keep the area clean and wash carefully, especially after the clips/sutures have been removed
- They are able to bathe immediately
- They may need to be off work for 6 weeks if their job involves lifting
- They should avoid prolonged coughing (control chronic obstructive pulmonary disease preoperatively)
- They should take laxatives if they get constipated postoperatively

ADVANCED QUESTIONS

(a) How would you perform a hernia repair?

Be prepared to discuss a method of hernia repair you have learned. The main points to remember are:

- Testicular damage should be mentioned as a specific risk-factor
- The operation can be performed under local or general anaesthetic and often as a day case
- The Royal College of Surgeons of England has recommended the Lichtenstein mesh repair and the Shouldice repair

(b) What are the complications of inguinal hernia repair?

Complications should be divided into *immediate* (first 24 hours), *early* (within the first month) and *late* (later than the first month) and further into *general* for any procedure and *specific* for this procedure.

Specific complications to mention:

- Urinary retention
- Bruising – occurs in 30%
- Pain – often very severe and patients should be discharged with adequate analgesia; chronic groin pain persists in 5% of patients
- Haematoma – 10%
- Infection – 1%
- Ischaemic orchitis – 0.5% (caused by thrombosis of the pampiniform plexus draining the testis)
  - previous vasectomy is a predisposing cause
  - dissection beyond (more medial than) the pubic tubercle is one operative risk and so this practice should be avoided
- Recurrence – should be < 0.5%
  - normally due to inadequate ring and posterior wall closure
  - occasionally due to overtight sutures

FURTHER READING

Cameron A E (1994) Accuracy of clinical diagnosis of direct and indirect inguinal hernia. *Br J Surg* **81**(2): 250.

McGreevy J M (1998) Groin hernia and surgical truth (editorial). *Am J Surg* **176**(4): 301–4.

Liem M S, van Vroonhoven T J (1996) Laparoscopic inguinal hernia repair. *Br J Surg* **83**(9): 1197–204.

www.gh.vic.gov.au\periop\abdo\inguinal.htm – gives information on what to tell patients about their inguinal hernia and what to expect from surgery

Differential diagnosis of a lump in the groin

Skin, soft tissues:

- Sebaceous cyst
- Lipoma

Vascular:

- Femoral artery aneurysm
- Sapheno varix
- Lymphadenopathy

Hernias:

- Inguinal
- Femoral

Renal/urogenital system:

- Ectopic or maldescended testis
- Transplanted kidney

CASE 43   ABDOMINAL EXAMINATION –   ***
GENERAL APPROACH

INSTRUCTION

'Examine this patient's abdomen.'

APPROACH

TOP TIP 1 – EXPOSURE OF THE ABDOMEN

The exposure of the abdomen is very important and opinions differ as to how much of the abdomen needs to be exposed (and at what point) during the clinical examination. Clearly, if there is an inguinal hernia or a scrotal lump, this will be missed if the external genitalia are not exposed. Equally, a patient who has an epigastric hernia should not have his or her dignity compromised.

You are not expected to say, 'I would expose the patient from nipple to knees'; this is both inappropriate to say in front of a patient and misses the point – that the degree of exposure depends on the case and how much the examiner expects of you.

We would advocate beginning by positioning the patient flat on the bed, but keep the groin covered until later on, starting your examination looking for peripheral stigmata of gastrointestinal disease.

VITAL POINTS

Inspect for peripheral stigmata of abdominal disease

Hands

- Take the patient's right hand and look for signs of chronic liver disease (*see* Case 46) and inflammatory bowel disease (*see* Case 50)
- Look for koilonychia (spoon-shaped nails in iron-deficiency anaemia) and pallor of the palmar creases in anaemia
- Check for a liver flap with both of the patient's hands (you can ask the patient to put his hands out in front of him and cock his wrists back as if he is stopping traffic) – in practice this is a late sign of hepatic encephalopathy and these patients will not be in examinations

Eyes

- Look in the eyes for anaemia (pale conjuctivae) and jaundice (*see* Case 14)

Mouth

- Look in the mouth (and smell) for oral manifestations of chronic gastrointestinal disease, e.g. hepatic foetor, pallor of the mucous membranes (*see* Case 72 for full description of mouth signs in abdominal disease)

Neck

- Palpate the neck for supraclavicular lymphadenopathy – Virchow's node (also known as Troisier's sign) is found in the supraclavicular fossa between the sternal and clavicular heads of the sternocleidomastoid muscle

Trunk

- Inspect the rest of the arms and upper chest wall for spider naevi, which are in the distribution of drainage of the superior vena cava (*see* Case 41)
- Briefly inspect the back, by asking the patient to roll towards and away from you

Expose the patient's abdomen

- If it is a man, ask them to remove their shirt
- If it is a woman, keep the bra on but expose the chest otherwise
- Expose down to the symphysis pubis, keeping the genitalia covered

Stand back from the couch

Stand at the end or to the side of the couch, and inspect the abdomen thoroughly, looking for:

- Distension
- Scars (*see* Case 62)
- Visible pulsation
- Ask the patient to take a deep breath in and hold it, seeing the transmitted pulsation of an abdominal aortic aneurysm
- Ask the patient to cough or lift their head off the bed, demonstrating any herniae – especially important if scars are present

Palpate

Kneel down next to the patient's right side and ask if they have any pain anywhere, before beginning to palpate the abdomen. Look at the patient's face the whole time when attempting to elicit any tenderness:

- Begin furthest away from you and palpate the nine quadrants of the abdomen with the four fingers of your right hand held together, first lightly, testing particularly for tenderness
- When you arrive in the epigastric region, *pause for pulsation*, testing for an abdominal aortic aneurysm (*see* Case 115)
- Continue with deep palpation in the same nine quadrants, feeling for any masses – often this is done using two hands interlocked above each other
- Palpate the liver (*see* Case 46) and spleen (*see* Case 49) in turn
- Attempt to ballot the kidneys (*see* Case 61)

Percuss

- If there is hepatosplenomegaly the spleen and liver should be percussed
- If there is any abdominal distension you should percuss for ascites (*see* Case 57)

Auscultate

- Over the liver for a bruit
- In the left iliac fossa for bowel sounds
- Over the abdominal aorta and iliac vessels for bruits

Continue

Continue if you have not found any abnormality by exposing the external genitalia and examining the scrotum (*see* Case 51) and inguinal canal for herniae (*see* Case 44). Palpate the femoral pulses and check for femoral herniae.

Finish your examination here

Make sure to cover the patient back up and ensure they are comfortable.

Completion

Complete the examination by telling the examiner you would:

- Review the observation chart (temperature, blood pressure, pulse and respiratory rate)
- Examine the lower limbs for peripheral oedema
- Examine the external genitalia and groin (if not already done)
- Perform a digital rectal examination
- Dipstick the urine

TOP TIP 2
The term 'per rectal' is vague; 'digital rectal examination' is more appropriate.

C. E. Troisier (1844–1919). Professor of Pathology, Paris. Also described haemachromatosis (Troisier syndrome).
R. L. K. Virchow (1821–1902). Professor of Pathology, Wurzberg and Berlin. Also described Virchow space (perivascular space of Virchow–Robin), Virchow cell (lepra cell) and the Virchow triad of thrombogenesis.

*** **SURGICAL JAUNDICE** **CASE 44**

INSTRUCTION 1

'Ask this patient some questions about her jaundice.'

APPROACH

Direct your questions to finding out whether the cause of her jaundice is likely to be pre-hepatic, hepatic or post-hepatic. Remember that in the surgical short case, post-hepatic is the most likely cause and this is the easiest to diagnose from the history:

- Have you noticed any change in the colour of your urine?
- Have you noticed any change in the colour of your stools?
- Have you noticed yourself feeling itchy?

If the patient has noticed pale stools and dark urine, then explore possible causes:

- Weight-loss, change in bowel habit, loss of appetite and back pain are associated with primary and secondary intra-abdominal malignancies
- Younger age, previous biliary colic or episodic right upper quadrant pains may indicate gallstones

Continue by asking some questions differentiating the other types of jaundice, and possibly to identify any risk-factors for hepatic jaundice, such as foreign travel (hepatitis A), blood transfusion (hepatitis B and C), sore throat (Epstein–Barr virus), alcohol intake, and use of certain drugs such as the oral contraceptive pill and phenothiazines.

INSTRUCTION 2

'Examine this lady's abdomen.'

APPROACH

Expose the patient as previously (Case 43) and begin by examining the hands.

VITAL POINTS

- Look for signs of chronic liver disease (*see* Case 46).
- Confirm the presence of jaundice by looking at the sclera (*see* TOP TIP)
- Examine the neck for Virchow's node (*see* Case 43)

Inspect

- The abdomen may be distended with ascites
- There may be distended veins around the umbilicus if there is portal hypertension (caput medusae – *see* Case 128)

> TOP TIP
>
> When examining the eyes for jaundice or anaemia, only look into one eye (the sign will be bilateral if present). It is easier to use your left thumb to lower the patient's lower eyelid and ask them to look towards the ceiling in order to get the best opportunity to inspect the sclera and conjuctiva.
>
> If you suspect a jaundiced sclera but you are unsure, continue to examine the patient's soft palate with a pen torch. Bilirubin is avidly taken up by tissues that are rich in elastin, and therefore the soft palate is a sensitive indicator of the presence of jaundice.

Palpate

- Palpate the abdomen as previously (*see* Case 43)
- Palpate carefully in the right upper quadrant identifying any tenderness or masses, remembering Courvoisier's law: *in the presence of obstructive jaundice a mass in the right upper quadrant is unlikely to be due to gallstones*

Finish your examination here

Completion

You would want to:

- Complete the abdominal examination (*see* Case 43) by checking the hernial orifices, examining the external genitalia, performing a digital rectal examination and examining the lower limbs for peripheral oedema
- Check the temperature to see whether the potential obstruction has been complicated by infection
- Dipstick the urine for raised levels of bilirubin

QUESTIONS

(a) How can jaundice be classified?

Jaundice is yellow discolouration of the skin and mucous membranes caused by the accumulation of bile pigments. The causes can be classified (*see* Table 14) into:

- Pre-hepatic
- Hepatic
- Post-hepatic

(b) What level does the serum bilirubin need to rise to before jaundice can be detected on clinical examination?

Normal bilirubin is < 17 μmol/l and it usually has to reach at least three times this before the sclera is discoloured (i.e. > 50 μmol/l). Very high levels of bilirubin are usually associated with hepatic jaundice.

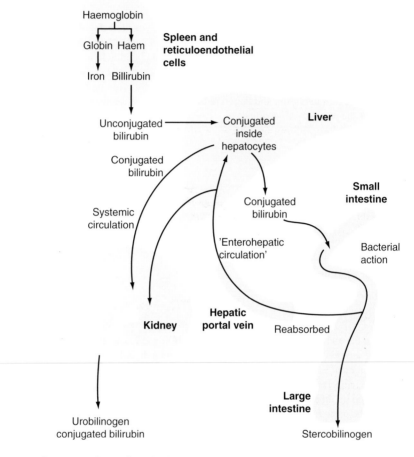

Fig. 16 Pathway for bilirubin excretion.

(c) Assuming this lady has obstructive jaundice, how should she be investigated?

Urine should be tested for raised bilirubin (see Fig. 16).
Blood tests:

- Full blood count – evidence of anaemia in GI malignancies or associated infection
- Renal function – any evidence of hepatorenal syndrome
- Liver function tests – see below
- Clotting – functional assessment of hepatic impairment

Radiological investigations:

- Ultrasound will show:
  - presence of underlying liver disease
  - degree of dilatation of the common bile duct (> 8 mm is abnormal)
  - presence of gall stones
  - presence of lymphadenopathy or a pancreatic mass
- Endoscopic retrograde cholangiopancreatography (ERCP)
- CT scan

(d) How might the liver function tests help in distinguishing the types of jaundice?

This is particularly important in OSCEs, where you may be asked to interpret liver function test results (Table 14).

Table 14   Causes of jaundice and effects on liver function tests

	Pre-hepatic	Hepatic	Post-hepatic

Major causes	Haemolysis
	Hereditary, e.g.
	   Gilbert's syndrome
		Hepatitis
		Decompensated
		   chronic liver
		   disease
		
		Drugs
			Gallstones
			Carcinoma head
			   of pancreas
			
			Lymph nodes

Bili type	Unconjugated	Conjugated	Conjugated
Bili increase	++	+++/++++	++
ALT	+/++	++/+++	+/++
ALP	-/+	+/++	++/+++

Bili = bilirubin; ALT = alanine aminotransferase (similar rises with aspartate aminotransferase, AST); ALP = alkaline phosphatase

ADVANCED QUESTIONS

(a) What are the causes of post-operative jaundice?

- Pre-hepatic jaundice can occur due to haemolysis, especially following a transfusion
- Hepatic jaundice can result from the use of halogenated anaesthetics, sepsis or intra- or post-operative hypotension
- Post-hepatic jaundice can occur due to biliary injury (such as in laparoscopic cholecystectomy)

> *Nicolas Augustin Gilbert (1858–1927).* French physician who worked on the classification of liver disease

FURTHER READING

http://www.nlm.nih.gov/medlineplus/ency/article/000210.htm – online medical encyclopaedia explaining the various causes of jaundice.

INSTRUCTION

'Inspect this lady's abdomen and comment on what you see.'

APPROACH

Expose the patient as in Case 43. Do not start at the hands as you have been given a specific direction to inspect the abdomen.

VITAL POINTS

Inspect

- Site (right iliac fossa, left iliac fossa, etc.) (see Fig. 17)
- Whether it is covered by a bag or whether the bag has been removed
- Appearance – if the bag has been removed then comment on:
  - mucosal lining – does it look healthy?
  - presence of a spout or flush with the skin
  - end (one opening) or loop (an afferent and efferent portion of bowel with one common opening or two separate openings)
- Contents – if there is a bag covering the stoma then describe the bag and comment on:
  - urine
  - formed stool
  - semi-formed or liquid stool

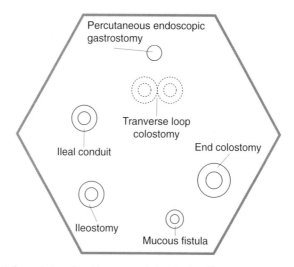

Fig. 17 Relevant sites for stomas on abdominal wall.

- Move on to describe the rest of the abdominal wall and remember there is likely to be a scar, which you should also describe (*see* Case 62)
- Are there any other drains/healed stoma sites?

Palpate

If you are only asked to inspect, then do not touch the patient at any time, even to move the stoma bag out of the way – there may be a good reason why you should not touch it

Finish your examination here

Completion

Tell the examiner you would continue to examine the rest of the abdomen to look for reasons why the stoma may have been formed in the first place.

QUESTIONS

(a) What are the indications for forming a stoma?

- Feeding, e.g. percutaneous endoscopic gastrostomy (PEG)
- Lavage, e.g. appendicostomy
- Decompression
- Diversion
  - 1. protect a distal bowel anastamosis
    - previously contaminated bowel
    - technical considerations – ileorectal anastamosis
  - 2. urinary diversion following cystectomy
- Exteriorization
  - perforated or contaminated bowel, e.g. distal abscess/fistula
  - permanent stoma, e.g. abdomino-perineal resection of rectum

(b) How would you prepare a patient who is going for surgery which will involve forming a stoma?

- Psychosocial and physical preparation
- Explanation of indications and complications
- This includes seeing a Clinical Nurse Specialist in Stoma Care preoperatively, who would normally mark the site
- Marking of the stoma site – *with the patient standing up* as he or she must be able to see the stoma
  - 5 cm from umbilicus
  - away from scars or skin creases
  - away from bony points or waistline of clothes
  - at a site that is easily accessible to the patient, e.g. not under a large fold of fat
- The stoma must be within the rectus abdominus sheath

(c) What are the complications of forming a stoma?

Complications can always be divided into specific to the procedure vs. general to any surgical procedure, and also into immediate (< 24 hours), early (< 1 month) and late (> 1 month).

Specific complications:

- Ischaemia/gangrene
- Haemorrhage
- Retraction
- Prolapse/intusussception
- Parastomal hernia
- Stenosis – leads to constipation
- Skin excoriation

General complications – related to underlying disease:

- Stoma diarrhoea – related to water and electrolyte imbalances, hypokalaemia being the commonest and most important consequence
- Nutritional disorders
- Stones – both gallstones and renal stones increase in frequency following an ileostomy
- Psychosexual
- Residual disease, e.g. Crohn's and parastomal fistula

(d) How can you tell the difference between an ileostomy and a colostomy?

See Table 15.

Table 15

	Ileostomy	Colostomy
Site	Right iliac fossa	Left iliac fossa
Surface	Spout (contents are corrosive and can damage local skin)	Flush with skin
Contents	Watery – small bowel content	Faeculent
Examples of permanent stomas	Post panproctocolectomy	Abdominoperoneal resection of rectum
Examples of temporary stomas	Loop ileostomy over low anastamosis of anterior resection	Hartmann's procedure (end colostomy)

(e) How would you rehabilitate a patient following the placement of a stoma?

- Diet should be normal
- Bag should be changed once or twice a day (needs to be emptied more frequently than this if it is urine or fluid faeces)
- Ileostomies should have the base plate under the bag changed every 5 days and the bag changed daily
- Psychological and psychosexual support

FURTHER READING

Shellito P C (1998) Complications of abdominal stoma surgery. *Dis Colon Rectum* **41**(12): 1562–72.

Cheung M T (1995) Complications of an abdominal stoma: an analysis of 322 stomas. *Aust N Z J Surg* **65**(11): 808–11.

www.bcass.org.uk – British Colostomy Association website – help and information for patients who are just about to have a colostomy.

CASE 46 HEPATOMEGALY ***

INSTRUCTION

'Examine this gentleman's abdomen.'

APPROACH

Expose the patient as per Case 43 and begin by examining the hands.

VITAL POINTS

Inspect

Look for the peripheral stigmata of chronic liver disease. In the hands:

- Digital clubbing – feature associated with cirrhosis of the liver, especially of primary biliary cirrhosis (*see also* Case 28)
- Leukonychia – 'white nails' associated with liver disease, fungal infection and can be congenital
- Terry's lines – white nails with normal pink tips seen in cirrhosis
- Palmar erythema – vasodilatation due to non-metabolized oestrogens
- Dupuytren's contracture – (*see* Case 78)
- Liver flap – ask the patient to hyperextend the hands, holding the arms straight out in front of them and cocking their wrists back 'as if you are trying to stop traffic' – look for flapping of the hands

In the rest of the arms, and upper trunk:

- Spider naevi
- Tattoos (risk-factor for transmission of hepatitis B and C virus)
- Scratch marks – icterus, or itch, is a sign of post-hepatic jaundice
- Gynaecomastia

In the face and neck:

- Pale conjunctiva
- Yellow sclera (*see* Case 44)
- Inside the mouth – smell for hepatic foetor
- Palpate the supraclavicular fossa for lymphadenopathy

Inspection of the abdomen

- The abdomen may be swollen due to ascites, and there might be a fullness in the right upper quadrant
- Note the presence of distended abdominal veins, which may occur in portal hypertension (caput medusae – *see* Case 128)

Examination of the liver

- Palpate the liver, beginning immediately above the right anterior superior iliac spine, in the right iliac fossa. Ask the patient to breathe in and move your hand proximally between each breath in order to detect the liver edge, coming down onto the hand in inspiration
- Define the distance in fingerbreadths from the costal margin at which the liver edge first appears
- Palpate the edge of the liver again, noting the presence of nodules and whether the edge is firm or smooth
- Percuss the upper edge of the liver, beginning at the top of the right hemithorax; the percussion note usually becomes dull at the level of the fifth rib
- At this point, auscultate the liver for a bruit (heard in hepatocellular carcinoma and alcoholic hepatitis)
- Check next for splenomegaly (*see* Case 49)
- Check for ascites if the abdomen is distended.

Finish your examination here

Completion

Tell the examiner you would:

- Complete the abdominal examination (*see* Case 43)
- Check for peripheral and sacral oedema (which occur in hypoalbuminaemia)

QUESTIONS

(a) How would you investigate this patient?

Blood tests:

- Full blood count – for example raised white cell count in infection
- Liver function – hypoalbuminaemia, evidence of hepatic dysfunction
- Clotting – functional hepatic impairment
- C-reactive protein/erythrocyte sedimentation rate – increased in infection/inflammation and in malignancy

Radiological investigations:

- Ultrasound is the first line radiological investigation – used to define the liver architecture, give an idea of the size and may identify the pathology
- Contrast-enhanced CT may also be useful, especially to further investigate solid lesions

(b) What are the causes of hepatomegaly?

Physiological:

- Reidel's lobe
- Hyperexpanded chest

Infections:

- Viral – viral hepatitis, Epstein–Barr virus, cytomegalovirus
- Bacterial – tuberculosis, liver abscess
- Protozoal – malaria, histoplasmosis, amoebiasis, hydatid, schistosomiasis

Alcoholic liver disease:

- Fatty liver (can also be caused by diabetes mellitus)
- Cirrhosis (other causes of cirrhosis also lead to hepatomegaly but these are less common)

Metabolic diseases:

- Wilson's disease
- Haemochromatosis
- Cellular infiltration, e.g. amyloid

Malignant disease:

- Primary/secondary solid tumours (secondary are more common)
- Lymphoma
- Leukaemia

Congestive cardiac disease:

- Right heart failure
- Tricuspid regurgitation (causes a pulsatile liver)
- Budd–Chiari syndrome

ADVANCED QUESTIONS

(a) What is the significance of an arterial bruit or venous hum over the liver?

An arterial bruit may indicate alcoholic hepatitis, and carcinoma. A venous hum is associated with portal hypertension and if this is secondary to cirrhosis with a patent umbilical vein (or varices in the falciform ligament), this is known as the Cruveilhier–Baumgarten syndrome.

(b) What is portal hypertension?

Defined as portal vein pressure of more than 10 mmHg (normal 5–10 mmHg). Portal blood flow through the liver is greatly reduced or even reversed in the most severe cases. The causes can broadly be divided into:

- Extrahepatic – caused by increased resistance to flow, e.g. portal or splenic vein thrombosis

- Intrahepatic – due to cirrhosis, right heart failure, sarcoidosis and schistosomiasis (the latter is the most important cause worldwide – ova of the parasite colonize and obstruct the portal venules)

> *W. Baumgarten (1873–1945).* Born in St Louis, Missouri, was one of founding members of the American Association of Physicians.
> *Jean Cruveilhier (1791–1874).* French pathologist, who also described gastric ulcers.
> *M. Epstein (1921–).* Professor of Pathology in Bristol, investigated Burkitt's lymphoma and identified this virus as important in its pathogenesis.
> *B. Riedel (1846–1916).* German surgeon and pathologist.
> *R. Terry.* British physician.

FURTHER READING

Garcia N Jr, Sanyal A J (2001) Portal hypertension. *Clin Liver Dis* **5**(2): 509–40.

www.british-liver-trust.org.uk – patient-centred website with information about viral hepatitis and regional liver support groups.

*** INCISIONAL HERNIA CASE 47

INSTRUCTION

'Examine this gentleman's abdomen.'

APPROACH

Begin the examination with the hands, but expect the examiner to move you straight to the exposure and examination of the abdomen itself.

VITAL POINTS

Inspect

- The patient may be overweight
- There will be a scar over the abdominal wall – describe the scar (*see* Case 62) and be sure to note the presence of any other scars, drain sites or old stomas
- Ask the patient to lift his head off the bed and note any bulging out of the scar
- Ask the patient to cough and, again, tell the examiner that you have demonstrated an element of weakness associated with the scar

Palpate

- Begin by palpating the patient's scar, asking whether there is any tenderness
- Note the presence of any nodularity and feel for the presence of a defect under all, or part of, the length of the incision
- Ask the patient to cough and feel the weakness in the scar allowing the intra-abdominal contents to come out into your hand
- Determine whether the defect is the whole length of the scar or not
- If the hernia was already present before the patient coughed (typically a very large defect), ask the patient whether he can push the lump back inside the abdomen

Auscultate

- Listen for bowel sounds if there is a large incarcerated hernia

Finish your examination here

Completion

Tell the examiner you would complete the rest of the abdominal examination, and wait to see whether he wants you to do so (implying there may be a second problem for you to identify)

QUESTIONS

(a) What is an incisional hernia?

- Extrusion of peritoneum and abdominal contents through a weak scar or accidental wound on the abdominal wall
- Represents a partial wound dehiscence where the skin remains intact

(b) What are the complications of incisional hernia?

- Intestinal obstruction (often intermittent)
- Incarceration and strangulation
- Skin excoriation
- Persistent pain

(c) What factors predispose to incisional hernia?

Preoperative:

- Age
- Immunocompromised state (including renal failure, diabetes, steroid use)
- Obesity
- Malignancy
- Abdominal distension from obstruction or ascites

Operative:

- Poor technical closure of the wound – using too small bites or inappropriate suture material
- Placing drains through wounds

Postoperative:

- Wound haematoma
- Wound infection
- Early mobilization
- Postoperative atelectasis and chest infection

ADVANCED QUESTIONS

(a) What are the treatment options for this patient?

Not every patient should undergo repair of his or her incisional hernia. Some patients will undergo operation and have a very high chance of wound haematoma and infection, dehiscence and recurrent hernia. In addition, many patients have concurrent medical problems (like obesity and chronic obstructive pulmonary disease) increasing their anaesthetic risk.

- Non-surgical:
  - use of a truss or corset
  - weight-loss and management of other risk-factors
- Surgical:
  - prior to surgery
    - cardiac and respiratory disease should be controlled first
    - other risk-factors should be optimized
    - preoperative weight-loss should be encouraged
  - surgical treatment principles are:
    - dissection of the hernial sac from surrounding tissues and definition of tissue bordering the defect on all sides to 2–3 cm
    - closing the defect and then using a mesh overlapping adequately over normal tissues to allow healing (about 3 cm) – now the technique of choice as it has been shown to be superior to suture repair
    - layered closure technique with sutures (especially if there is no tissue-loss)
    - large hernia may require the placing of postoperative drains

FURTHER READING

Khaira H S, Lall P, Hunter B, Brown J H (2001) Repair of incisional hernias. *J R Coll Surg Edinb* **46**(1): 39–43.

Luijendijk R W, Hop W C, van den Tol M P, *et al.* (2000). A comparison of suture repair with mesh repair for incisional hernia. *N Engl J Med* **343**(6): 392–8.

www.philly.com/content/inquirer/2001/09/03/magazine/DRH03.html – a North American surgeon answers patients questions about the reasons for operating on incisional hernias.

CASE 48   UMBILICAL HERNIA   * * *

INSTRUCTION

'Examine this gentleman's abdomen.'

APPROACH

Expose the patient and begin to examine the hands, as in Case 43, but expect the examiner to move you on.

VITAL POINTS

Inspect

- The patient may be overweight
- From the side or end of the couch ask the patient to lift his head off the bed and then to cough noticing the bulge appearing around or above the umbilicus
- Note any associated ulceration or skin damage
- Note the presence of an overlying scar indicating a recurrent hernia
- Point out the presence of a lump underlying the umbilicus, pushing the umbilicus out from the abdominal wall

Palpate

- Try to determine the size of the defect
- If there is a lump, ask the patient to 'push it back in' (do not attempt to do this yourself – they may be irreducible because loops of adherent omentum divide the sac into multilocular cavities)
- Ask the patient to cough, demonstrating an expansile cough impulse

Finish your examination here

Completion

Tell the examiner you would continue with the rest of the abdominal system examination.

QUESTIONS

(a) What is the pathogenesis of umbilical herniae?

These are due to a defect through the linea alba (the union of the rectus sheath in the midline) adjacent to the umbilicus and usually due to obesity stretching the fibres.

They are uncommon before the age of 40 years, but can grow to an enormous size. Peristalsis can be observed through the skin when the defect is large.

The neck of the sac is often tight and held with a fibrous band – this increases the rate of strangulation and infarction of contained bowel. Occasionally spontaneous discharge of the contents (as an enterocutanous fistula) can occur.

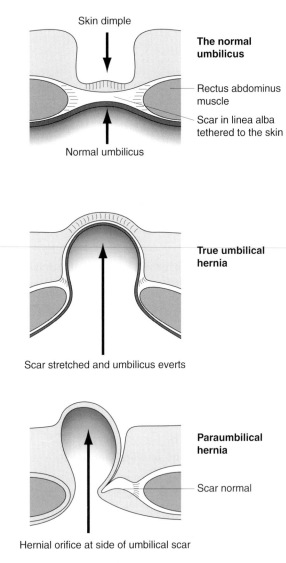

Skin dimple

The normal umbilicus

Rectus abdominus muscle

Scar in linea alba tethered to the skin

Normal umbilicus

True umbilical hernia

Scar stretched and umbilicus everts

Paraumbilical hernia

Scar normal

Hernial orifice at side of umbilical scar

Fig. 18   Umbilical and paraumbilical herniae.

(b) Tell me about umbilical herniae in children.

Minor defects in neonates are common but usually repair spontaneously. In older children, umbilical herniae are more common; they tend to have a narrow neck and folds of peritoneum stuck within this neck, which can occasionally strangulate. Most cases resolve before puberty and should only be repaired in symptomatic children.

(c) What differences are there in adults?

Acquired umbilical herniae may be caused by:

- Pregnancy
- Ascites
- Ovarian cysts
- Fibroids
- Bowel distension

They more commonly require surgical repair.

ADVANCED QUESTIONS

(a) How would this hernia be repaired?

It is important to mention the importance of treating concurrent medical problems prior to surgery; many of these patients have significant co-morbidity, which increases their anaesthetic risk. Where possible, the hernia should be repaired as the risk of strangulation is high.

Surgical technique – Mayo's 'vest-over-pants' operation is the most widely accepted repair for these herniae:

- A horizontal ellipse of stretched supra or infra-umbilical skin is excised, deepening the incision to the rectus sheath and identifying the fibrous band which is the neck of the sac
- The sac is opened near to the neck, returning protruding bowel to the abdomen
- The whole sac is removed
- The lower edge of the rectus is sutured behind the upper edge, so that the two flaps overlap using interrupted mattress absorbable sutures
- Often a mesh is used in large defect herniae

> *Charles Horace Mayo (1865–1939)* and *William James Mayo (1861–1939).*
> Brothers who founded the Mayo Clinic in Rochester, Minnesota.

FURTHER READING

Skinner M A, Grosfeld J L (1993). Inguinal and umbilical hernia repair in infants and children. *Surg Clin North Am* **73**(3): 439–49.

*** **SPLENOMEGALY** CASE 49

INSTRUCTION

'Examine this gentleman's abdomen.'

APPROACH

Expose the patient as for the abdominal examination (*see* Case 43).

VITAL POINTS

Peripheral stigmata

- Anaemia (pale nail bed, skin folds, mucous membranes)
- Lymphadenopathy
- There may also be stigmata of rheumatoid disease (*see* Case 80)

Inspect

- A fullness underneath the left costal margin may be seen

Palpate and percuss

Begin palpating for the spleen at the right iliac fossa (i.e. to the right of and below the umbilicus), moving your fingers towards the costal margin on the left hand side as the patient breathes in each time. The spleen is palpable below the costal margin on the left. Characteristically:

- You cannot 'get above' the spleen
- It moves with respiration
- It is dull to percussion (remember that the spleen underlies ribs 9–11 and while you are remembering that fact, note also that it is $1 \times 3 \times 5$ inches in size and that it weighs 7 oz, i.e. $1 \times 3 \times 5 \times 7 \times 9$–11)
- A notch may be palpable on the superomedial edge
- As it enlarges, it moves in the direction of the umbilicus
- It cannot be balloted (compared with an enlarged kidney)

TOP TIP

If the spleen is difficult to palpate, reach your left hand around the lower left rib cage and lift forwards as the patient breathes in – this manoeuvre may make a slightly enlarged spleen more easily palpable

---

Finish your examination here

Completion

Say that you would like to:

- Examine the rest of the abdomen particularly for hepatomegaly
- Listen to the heart for murmurs, and examine for other stigmata of infective endocarditis
- Enquire about foreign travel and symptoms of possible haematological malignancy

QUESTIONS

(a) What are the causes of splenomegaly?

Infective:

- Acute: Epstein–Barr virus, cytomegalovirus, HIV, infective endocarditis
- Chronic: toxoplasmosis, malaria, brucella, leishmaniasis, schistosomiasis

Haematological disease:

- Haemolytic anaemia
- Myeloproliferative disorders (especially myelofibrosis)
- Sickle cell disease/thalassaemia
- Leukaemia (especially chronic myeloid leukaemia, CML)
- Lymphoma

Portal hypertension:

- Cirrhosis
- Hepatic, portal or splenic vein thrombosis

Systemic diseases:

- Amyloidosis
- Sarcoidosis
- Rheumatoid arthritis (also remember Felty's syndrome – see below)

(b) What are the causes of massive splenomegaly?

- Myelofibrosis
- Chronic myeloid leukaemia
- Malaria
- Tropical splenomegaly
- Kala-azar (visceral leishmaniasis)

(c) What are the indications for splenectomy?

- Trauma
- Hypersplenism:
    - autoimmune thrombocytopaenia/haemolytic anaemia
    - hereditory spherocytosis
    - thrombotic thrombocytopaenia

– sickle cell/thalassaemia
– myelofibrosis, occasionally in CML, Hodgkin's

ADVANCED QUESTIONS

(a) What are the functions of the spleen?

- Produces IgM, to capture and process foreign antigen
- Filters especially capsulated microorganisms, e.g. pneumococcus
- Sequesters and removes old red blood cells and platelets
- Recycles iron
- Pools platelets (30% of total platelets within spleen)

(b) What immunizations would you need to organize in the event of performing a splenectomy?

Protocol depends on local guidelines but essentially:

- Pneumococcal vaccine
- *Haemophilis Influenzae* Type B vaccine
- Meningococcal vaccine
- Annual 'flu' vaccine
- Consideration for lifelong penicillin or penicillin as required when infection present
- Warn about risk of malaria, especially *Plasmodium falciparum*

(c) What are the appearances of the blood film after a splenectomy?

- Increased platelet count and large platelets
- Increased neutrophils
- Nucleated red cells with Howell–Jolly bodies and target cells
- Tend to mount more of a leukocytosis in response to infection

> *Augustus Roi Felty (1895–1963).* American physician who described the combination of splenomegaly, lymphadenopathy and leucopenia.

FURTHER READING

Baccarani U, Donini A, Terrosu G, Pasqualucci A, Bresadola F (1999) Laparoscopic splenectomy for haematological diseases: review of current concepts and opinions. *Eur J Surg* **165**(10): 917–23.

Glasgow R E and Mulvihill S J (1999) Laparoscopic splenectomy. *World J Surg* **23**(4): 384–8.

Farid H, O'Connell T X (1996) Surgical management of massive splenomegaly. *Am Surg* **62**(10): 803–5.

http://www.ssat.com/guidelines/spleen7.htm – patient care guidelines on splenectomy.

http://www.laparoscopy.net/spleen.htm – a guide to laparoscopic splenectomy.

CASE 50   INFLAMMATORY BOWEL DISEASE   ***

INSTRUCTION

'Examine this lady's abdomen.'

APPROACH

Expose the patient as in Case 43 and begin by examining the hands.

VITAL POINTS

Inspect for peripheral stigmata of gastrointestinal disease

- General signs of malnutrition or weight-loss
- In the hands, look for:
  - digital clubbing
  - pale skin creases if anaemic
- In the eyes look for:
  - pale conjunctivae if anaemic, uveitis, iritis, episcleritis
- Around the mouth look for:
  - aphthous ulceration, often severe, deep ulcers
- If the patient is an inpatient, comment on the:
  - intravenous lines, blood transfusions and fluids
  - central venous pressure line
  - urinary catheter

Inspect abdominal signs

Comment on all the signs on the abdominal wall, including:

- Scars (*see* Case 62) – in cases of complicated Crohn's disease these may be multiple, and not typical – just describe the anatomical location of each scar
- Stomas (*see* Case 45) or healed stoma sites
- Enterocutaneous fistulae (more common in Crohn's disease)
- Abdominal drains or healed drain sites

Palpate

- In acute exacerbations the abdomen may be distended and tense
- There may be a mass, most commonly in the right iliac fossa (*see* Case 55)
- Note the site of any tenderness
- The patient may have hepatomegaly

Percuss

If the abdomen is distended the percussion note is likely to be hyper-resonant.

Auscultate

Bowel sounds may be increased in acute exacerbations – likely to be normal in the exam itself.

Finish your examination here

Completion

Tell the examiner you would complete the abdominal system examination as in Case 43 (inspection of the perineum and the digital rectal examination is particularly important), and that you would examine for regional manifestations of Crohn's disease:

- Large joint mono-arthritis and sacroiliitis
- Pyoderma gangrenosum
- Erythema nodosum (usually over the extensor surfaces of the limbs)

QUESTIONS

(a) What investigations would you perform?

Stool tests:

- A stool culture should be performed in cases of exacerbation of inflammatory bowel disease as there may be an infective element

Blood tests:

- Full blood count may show anaemia and leukocytosis
- Electrolytes may show evidence of dehydration, or hypokalaemia
- Liver function tests
- C-reactive protein and erythrocyte sedimentation rate may be raised, which can also be used to monitor progress of the disease

Endoscopy:

- A sigmoidoscopy and biopsy would be indicated

Radiology:

- Depending on the exact symptoms a barium enema or small bowel study might be required

(b) What is the definition of severe exacerbation of inflammatory bowel disease?

Local symptoms:

- Passage of stool > 10 times per day
- Passage of blood with each stool
- Urge to defaecate
- Abdominal pain and distension

Systemic signs:

- Tachycardia
- Pyrexia
- Pallor
- Wasting

(c) What are the indications for surgery in exacerbations of inflammatory bowel disease?

- Toxic megacolon (transverse diameter of colon of at least 6 cm on a plain abdominal X-ray) – high risk of perforation and faecal peritonitis
- Failure of medical management to control symptoms
- Intestinal fistulae
- Intra-abdominal abscesses that cannot be drained radiologically
- Entero-cutaneous fistulae (but see notes in Case 71)
- Presence of dysplasia on colonoscopic biopsies
- Development of carcinoma
- Complications of long-term steroid use

ADVANCED QUESTIONS

(a) What are the hepatobiliary complications of inflammatory bowel disease?

Liver:

- Fatty change
- Chronic active hepatitis
- Cirrhosis
- Amyloid deposition

Gall bladder and bile ducts:

- Gallstones
- Sclerosing cholangitis
- Cholangiocarcinoma

(b) What are the surgical options for managing ulcerative colitis?

Proctocolectomy and permanent ileostomy (= panproctocolectomy):

- Rectum and anus excised with all of the colon
- Indicated for carcinoma or dysplasia, and failed medical management

Sub-total colectomy, mucous fistula and permanent ileostomy:

- Rectum brought out as a mucous fistula and an ileostomy formed in the right iliac fossa
- Further rectal symptoms can occur in the mucous fistula but these can usually be controlled with topical agents
- Indicated for toxic megacolon

Restorative proctocolectomy:

- Three-stage procedure which removes the need for a permanent ileostomy
- Neo-rectum is created in a pelvic reservoir
- Stage 1: subtotal colectomy and end ileostomy
- Stage 2: residual rectum has mucosa removed and the pouch is placed within a tube of rectal muscle, anastamosed to the anus – this is covered with a defunctioning loop ileostomy
- Stage 3: contrast radiology demonstrated intact pouch and the loop ileostomy is reversed

(c) What are the surgical options for Crohn's disease?

- In surgery for the small intestine, as much bowel should be left after the operation as possible
- Intra-abdominal abscesses should be drained
- Colonic dysfunctioning using a loop ileostomy may be needed for patients who have failed medical therapy
- Occasionally a subtotal colectomy and permanent end ileostomy may be needed
- Pouch surgery is contraindicated in Crohn's disease

> *Burrell Bernard Crohn (born 1884).* US physician working in New York who became the president of the American Gastroenterology Society, presenting a paper in 1932 which described Crohn's disease.

FURTHER READING

www.nacc.org.uk – website of the UK national association for colitis and Crohn's disease, a charity for patients with inflammatory bowel disease

CASE 51   EXAMINATION OF THE SCROTUM –   **
GENERAL APPROACH

INSTRUCTION

'Examine this gentleman's scrotum.'

APPROACH

It is important to listen to the stem of the question, as there will be a clue as to whether the problem is in the groin or in the scrotum itself. If asked to examine the groin then begin with the inguinal hernia examination (*see* Case 42), unless there is an obvious mass or swelling in the hemiscrotum.

If the patient is lying on a bed then examine him supine, remembering to ask him to stand up at the end to ensure that you do not miss a varicocele. If he is standing or sitting in a chair, then examine him standing.

VITAL POINTS

Inspect

The key distinction in these cases is whether the problem arises from the groin (is it an indirect inguinoscrotal hernia?) or is of scrotal origin:

- Inspect the groin and scrotum
- Scrotal incisions may be difficult to see as they are frequently made in the median raphe in between the two hemiscrotums
- Check in the groins, identifying any oblique groin incisions, which may have been used to approach the testes

Palpate

Ask the patient if he has any pain and watch his face while palpating the scrotum:

- Palpate both testes, one at a time
- When palpating the testis, place the fingers of one hand behind the testis, supporting it, while examining the surface of the testis with the thumb
- Palpate the normal contour of the testis, identifying the epididymis and the ductus deferens as well
- The surface of the testis is normally firm and regular
- Lumps and irregularity, and especially any hard masses, are abnormal and should precipitate further investigation

Lumps in the groin can easily be distinguished by answering a few key questions (*see* Cases 52, 53, 54 and 70 for details):

- Is the lump separate from the testis, i.e. can you identify the testis and epididymis?
- Can you get above it?
- Does it transilluminate?

Finish your examination here

Completion

- Tell the examiner you would continue to examine the rest of the abdomen and groin (see specific cases)
- The lymph drainage of the testes are to the para-aortic nodes which are retroperitoneal and unless extremely large will not be palpable
- Inguinal lymphadenopathy is not likely to be a response of testicular problems, but the lymph drainage from the skin of the scrotum and penis is to the inguinal nodes, and if there is pathology involving the scrotal skin or a squamous cell carcinoma of the penis, then these nodes may be enlarged

** HYDROCELE   CASE 52

INSTRUCTION

'Examine this gentleman's scrotum.'

APPROACH

See Case 51.

VITAL POINTS

Inspect

The scrotum may be very swollen if the hydrocele is large.

Palpate

The mass is:
- Usually inseparable from the testis (although a hydrocele of the cord will be separate) and uniformly enlarged
- Firm – may be tense or lax
- May be transilluminable (tends to transluminate less as it becomes more chronic)
- Distinct from the superficial inguinal ring (you can 'get above' the mass)

Hydroceles vary enormously in size and some patients who come along to examinations have chronic hydroceles which may be very large – it may be that some other medical problem makes surgical intervention hazardous

Finish your examination here

Completion

Always remember to examine the contralateral scrotum.

QUESTIONS

(a) What is a hydrocele?

Excess accumulation of fluid in the processus vaginalis. During the descent of the testis from the posterior abdominal wall *in utero*, it carries a fold of peritoneum, the processus vaginalis. This normally forms the tunica vaginalis, one of the adult coverings of the testis, and the rest of the connection from the abdomen is obliterated. Should this obliteration not occur, and fluid accumulate in any part of this peritoneum-derived covering, a hydrocele forms.

(b) What is the anatomical classification hydroceles?

- Vaginal hydrocele – fluid accumulates in the tunica vaginalis which surrounds the testis but does not extend up into the cord
- Hydrocele of the cord – fluid accumulates around the spermatic cord and therefore the mass appears around the ductus deferens. This may be very difficult to distinguish from an irreducible inguinal hernia, as it may extend up to and beyond the superficial inguinal ring into the groin. If in doubt, traction on the testis causes a hydrocele of the cord to be pulled downwards
- Congenital hydrocele – the proximal part of the processus vaginalis has not obliterated, the sac communicates directly with the peritoneum and the hydrocele is filled with peritoneal fluid
- Infantile hydrocele – a situation in between the congenital hydrocele and hydrocele of the cord; the processus vaginalis is obliterated at the deep ring and so the hydrocele does not communicate with the abdomen but it remains patent in both the cord and scrotum

ADVANCED QUESTIONS

(a) What are the treatment options?

Non-surgical:

- 'Watch and wait' – a small hydrocele may require no treatment other than reassurance, but an underlying malignancy should be excluded (clinically and with an ultrasound)
- Aspiration – the hydrocele fluid can be aspirated to relieve symptoms; tends to reaccumulate

Surgical:

- Lord's plication – small incision through the scrotum to lift out the testis; the sac is plicated with a series of interrupted sutures to the junction of the testis and epididymis
- Jaboulay's operation – the sac is everted through a longitudinal incision, excess sac is excised and the remainder replaced behind the cord

(b) What is a secondary hydrocele?

Although most hydroceles are the result of a patent processus vaginalis, the vaginal type can be secondary to a number of local pathologies:

- Testicular tumours
- Torsion
- Orchitis
- Trauma
- Following inguinal hernia repair

> *Peter Lord.* Contemporary surgeon at Wycombe General Hospital, England, also named the 'Lord's stretch', for treatment of anal fissure, and 'Lord's directors', instruments used to assist knot-tying within the abdominal cavity.

FURTHER READING

Davenport M (1996) ABC of general paediatric surgery. Inguinal hernia, hydrocele, and the undescended testis. *BMJ* **312**(7030): 564–7.

** ** **EPIDIDYMAL CYST**   **CASE 53**

INSTRUCTION

'Examine this gentleman's scrotum.'

APPROACH

As in Case 51.

VITAL POINTS

Inspect

- Unless the cyst is unusually large the scrotum will appear normal

Palpate

The mass is:
- Separate from the testis – within the epididymis
- Firm, and may be loculated
- May be brilliantly transilluminable, unless they contain sperm in which case they do not transilluminate (this description is classical but can only be demonstrated in large cysts)
- Distinct from the superficial inguinal ring (you can 'get above' the mass)

Finish your examination here

Completion

Remember to examine the contralateral hemiscrotum.

QUESTIONS

(a) How are epididymal cysts caused?

They are often multiple and most commonly arise in the head of the epididymis. Occasionally they occur as a complication of vasectomy, in which case they are full of sperm and are termed spermatoceles.

(b) How should they be managed?

Non-surgical:

- If the cyst is not troublesome it should not be removed, especially in younger men, because there is risk of operative damage and postoperative fibrosis causing subfertility

Surgical:

- Very large or painful cysts can be removed and occasionally excision of the entire epididymis is indicated to prevent frequent recurrence of painful cysts.

FURTHER READING

http://www.surgerydoor.co.uk/tiscali/so/detail2.asp?level2=Epididymal%20Cyst %20Removal – information for patients on how an epididymal cyst is removed.

CASE 54	VARICOCELE ★★

INSTRUCTION

'Examine this gentleman's scrotum.'

APPROACH

As in Case 51.

VITAL POINTS

Inspect

The scrotum will usually appear normal but the testis on the side of the varicocele may hang lower than the other side

Palpate

The varicocele does not usually appear until the patient is standing up; all scrotal examinations should include an examination of the patient standing to exclude a varicocele. Ask the patient to cough while palpating the varicocele

The mass is characterized by:

- Being separate from the testis
- 'Bag of worms' feel
- Non-transilluminable
- Distinct from the superficial inguinal ring (you can 'get above' the mass)
- May have a palpable cough impulse

Finish your examination here

Completion

Remember to examine the contralateral hemiscrotum.

QUESTIONS

(a) What is the aetiology of varicoceles?

- Varicoceles are dilated tortuous 'varicose' veins in the pampiniform plexus, the network of veins that drains the testis (draining eventually into the testicular vein)
- They usually occur in up to 15% of younger men, often around puberty, and are thought to have an anatomical basis
- If they appear suddenly in older men, underlying retroperitoneal disease should be sought, including renal carcinoma extending into the left renal vein – clinically these may be suggested by varicoceles that do not disappear on lying supine

ADVANCED QUESTIONS

(a) Why are 98% of varicoceles left-sided?

- The left spermatic vein is more vertical where it connects to the left renal vein
- The left renal vein can be compressed by the colon
- The left testicular vein is longer than the right
- It frequently lacks a terminal valve which serves to try to prevent back-flow in the vein

(b) What are the treatment options?

Non-surgical:

- Transfemoral radiological embolization of the testicular vein, using either a spring coil or sclerosant

Surgical:

- Surgical treatment is often advised as the problem usually gets worse with age and there is a risk of infertility
- Palomo operation – exposure of the testicular artery by the high retroperitoneal approach, through an incision above and medial to the anterior superior iliac spine and ligation of all the surrounding veins
- Inguinal approach – similar principle with ligation of the veins in the inguinal canal
- Laparoscopic ligation is also possible

FURTHER READING

Jarow J P (2001) Effect of varicocele on male fertility. *Hum Reprod Update* **7**(1): 59–64.

Cornud F, Belin X, Amar E, Delafontaine D, Helenon O, Moreau J F (1999) Varicocele: strategies in diagnosis and treatment. *Eur Radiol* **9**(3): 536–45.

www.netdoctor.co.uk/diseases/facts/hydrocele – review of both hydrocele and varicocele.

CASE 55   RIGHT ILIAC FOSSA MASS   **

INSTRUCTION

'Examine this lady's abdomen.'

APPROACH

Expose the patient and begin, as in Case 43, by examining the hands.

VITAL POINTS

Inspect peripheral signs

In the hands look for:

- Digital clubbing (inflammatory bowel disease)
- Pale skin creases (anaemia, e.g. chronic bleeding from colonic carcinoma)
- Arteriovenous fistula at the wrist (transplanted kidney)

In the eyes look for:

- Pale conjunctivae (anaemia)
- Sclera (jaundice)

In the neck, palpate:

- Lymphadenopathy, especially noting the presence of a Virchow's node in the left supraclavicular fossa (Case 43)

Inspect abdominal signs

Note the presence of any scars from previous surgery and asymmetry may suggest an abdominal mass – especially note the presence of scars indicating renal transplantation (*see* Case 56)

Palpate

Begin palpating the abdomen as in Case 43. When you locate the mass, differentiate the mass before continuing with the rest of the abdominal examination. Note the:

- Size
- Edge – well defined or poorly defined
- Surface – smooth/irregular/nodular
- Relations – does it arise from the pelvis or are you able to place a hand between the pelvis and the mass
- Attachment to skin
- Attachment to the abdominal wall muscles – ask the patient to lift their head up off the bed while palpating the mass

Finish your examination here

Completion

Further examination would depend on your diagnosis but would include completing the rest of the abdominal system examination.

QUESTIONS

(a) What are the causes of a mass in the right iliac fossa?

The best way to classify this answer is to think of the different anatomical layers and structures within the right iliac fossa – this avoids leaving out any important causes.

Arising from the skin and soft tissues:
- Sebaceous cyst
- Lipoma
- Sarcoma

Arising from the bowel:
- Carcinoma of the caecum
- Crohn's mass in the terminal ileum
- Tuberculosis of the terminal ileum
- Appendicular mass or abscess

Arising from the gynaecological system:
- Ovarian tumours (benign and malignant)
- Fibroid uterus

Arising from the male reproductive system:
- Incompletely descended testis (Fig. 19)
- Ectopic testis (Fig. 20)

Arising from the urological system:
- Transplanted kidney
- Ectopic kidney
- Bladder diverticulum

Arising from blood vessels:
- External iliac or common iliac artery aneurysm
- Lymphadenopathy

(b) What radiological investigations would be helpful in distinguishing the possible causes?

- Ultrasound would be the first investigation – this would distinguish a bowel mass from an ovarian or uterine mass, and would identify any lymph nodes or abnormal blood vessels
- Abdominal wall masses are better seen with CT scan, and this would also be useful in looking at the extent of intra-abdominal malignant disease
- Intravenous contrast-enhanced CT scanning would clarify lower abdominal and pelvic vasculature

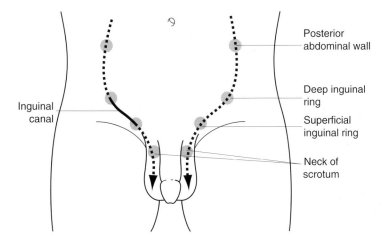

Fig. 19 Incompletely descended testis.

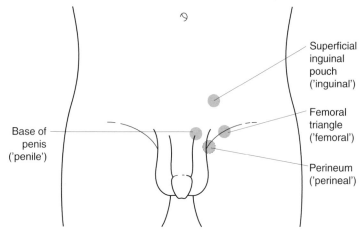

Fig. 20   Ectopic testis.

Differential diagnosis of a mass in the left iliac fossa

This is a very similar list to the one above; the only change is in the 'arising from the bowel' section:

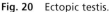

- Diverticular mass (often tender)
- Carcinoma of the colon
- Faecal mass

**   TRANSPLANTED KIDNEY   **CASE 56**

INSTRUCTION

'Examine this gentleman's abdomen.'

APPROACH

Expose the patient as in Case 43 and begin by examining the hands.

VITAL POINTS

Inspect peripheral signs

- There may be signs of anaemia (pale palmar skin creases, pale conjunctiva)
- A scar may be visible over the wrist at the site of a Bresica–Cimino arteriovenous fistula (*see* Case 131).
- There may be signs of steroid use (e.g. bruising, thin skin)

Inspect the abdomen

- Note the swelling in the right or left iliac fossa
- There will be a specific scar over the iliac fossa; a curved inguinal incision is used to perform the transplant (a Rutherford–Morrison incision)
- Note also the presence of previous nephrectomy scars and points of access of old dialysis catheters

Palpate

Note the mass in the right or left iliac fossa – the mass is superficial and well defined as the transplanted kidney is placed outside the peritoneum, covered only by the external and internal oblique and transversus abdominus muscles. It should only be palpated very lightly.

Finish your examination here

QUESTIONS

(a) What are the major indications for renal transplantation?

Renal transplantation is indicated in end stage renal failure, the commonest reasons in the UK are:

- Diabetes mellitus
- Hypertensive renal disease
- Glomerulonephritis
- Polycystic kidney disease

ADVANCED QUESTIONS

(a) How is 'matching' of transplanted kidneys performed?

Matching is performed at two levels:

- ABO compatability
- HLA compatability, matching at the HLA-DR locus has the greatest importance followed by matching at the HLA-B locus and then at the HLA-A locus

In patients who are HLA and ABO matched the 1-year donor kidney survival rate is 90%. Blood transfusions prior to transplant should be avoided as this carries the risk of HLA sensitization.

(b) What occurs in 'transplant rejection'?

Rejection is genetically modified and also relates to HLA incompatability. It can be divided into:

- Hyperacute – within hours of surgery – due to pre-formed antibodies in a sensitized recipient
- Accelerated acute – 1 to 4 days postoperatively – due to a 'secondary immune response' as a consequence of activation of memory T cells
- Acute – 5 days to 2 weeks after surgery – cell-mediated immunity related; renal epithelial cells are destroyed by a lymphocyte interstitial infiltrate

- Chronic – humoral mechanisms more important, tubular atrophy and interstitial fibrosis are the histological features

(c) How might you be aware that transplant rejection is occurring?

The features that may be expected are:

- Tenderness over the graft
- Reduction in urine output
- Rising creatinine

(d) Describe the vascular supply of the transplanted kidney

- The donor renal artery is anastamosed to either the internal or external iliac artery (Fig. 21)
- The donor renal vein is reattached to the external iliac vein
- The ureter is attached separately to the patient's bladder
- The renal pelvis is the most anterior structure, then artery and the vein most posterior

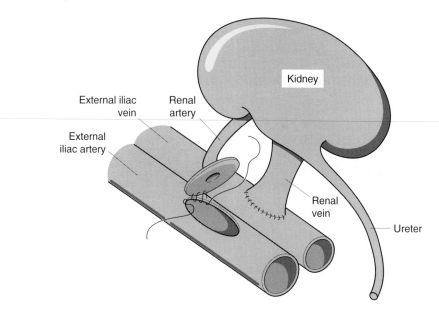

Fig. 21 Vascular supply of the transplanted kidney.

FURTHER READING

Paduch D A, Barry J M, Arsanjani A and Lemmers M J (2001) Indication, surgical technique and outcome of orthotopic renal transplantation. *J Urol* **166**(5): 1647–50.

Tejani A and Emmett L (2001) Acute and chronic rejection. *Semin Nephrol* **21**(5): 498–507.

CASE 57 ASCITES ★ ★

INSTRUCTION

'Examine this gentleman's abdomen.'

APPROACH

Expose the patient and begin to examine the abdomen as in Case 43.

VITAL POINTS

Inspect

- The abdomen may be distended if the ascites is gross – distension will tend to be lateral, as fluid accumulates in the paracolic gutters when the patient is supine
- Begin at the hands, noting any peripheral stigmata of chronic liver disease (*see* Case 46)

Specific tests for ascites

- Flank dullness – percussion over the flanks is dull because of accumulated fluid in the paracolic gutters
- Shifting dullness – define the margin where the percussion note first becomes dull in the left flank; then ask the patient to roll towards you, keeping your finger on the same point on the abdomen, wait for the fluid to resettle and then demonstrate the percussion note has become resonant again
- Fluid thrill – with large volumes of ascites, a transmitted thrill can be felt. Ask the patient to place his hand parallel to the body over the umbilicus, resting firmly on the abdomen (Fig. 22). Tap gently with your left hand onto his right flank, feeling the transmitted pulsation with your right hand resting on the left flank.

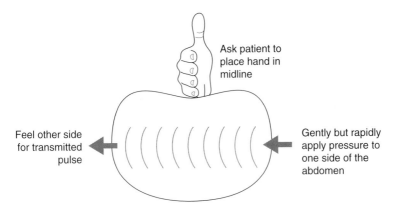

Ask patient to place hand in midline

Feel other side for transmitted pulse

Gently but rapidly apply pressure to one side of the abdomen

Fig. 22 Fluid thrill.

Finish your examination here

> **TOP TIP**
>
> It can be extremely difficult to palpate the liver in patients with ascites. If possible, percuss the abdomen for fluid before continuing to examine for organomegaly – the examiner may stop you at this point.

Completion

Tell the examiner you would:

- Examine the rest of the abdomen looking for other problems, and in particular evidence of intra-abdominal malignancy
- Continue to look for ankle and sacral oedema (signs of hypoalbuminaemia)
- Examine the chest for signs of right heart failure

QUESTIONS

(a) What are the causes of ascites?

Common:

- Chronic liver disease
- Right heart failure
- Intra-abdominal malignancy
- Hypoalbuminaemia

Uncommon:

- Nephrotic syndrome
- Tuberculosis
- Chylous ascites

ADVANCED QUESTIONS

(a) How would you perform an ascitic tap?

The procedure should be performed under sterile conditions and if the ascites is not clinically apparent or easy to locate, it should be done by a radiologist under ultrasound guidance to prevent inadvertent injuries to intra-abdominal structures:

- Local anaesthetic is infiltrated and the site marked
- A narrow-gauge needle should be introduced first to check the position before a larger-gauge cannula is inserted into the abdomen
- When in position, a plastic tube can be connected to a urine bag in order to collect the ascitic fluid from the abdominal cavity

- Samples of fluid are taken for
  - cytology (presence of any malignant cells)
  - protein (difference between exudate and transudate – an exudate has protein content of > 30 g/l)
  - microbiology (to exclude bacterial peritonitis as a complication)

(b) With which conditions would an exudate be expected?

See Table 16.

Table 16

Transudate (Protein < 30 g/l)	Exudate (Protein > 30 g/l)
Cardiac failure	Cirrhosis
Tricuspid regurgitation	Malignancy
Constrictive pericarditis	Lymphatic rupture or damage

(c) What are the indications for the use of a shunt in the management of ascites?

The mainstay of treatment of ascites is to treat the underlying condition and to place the patient on a weight reduction program, with the help of diuretics, and a low-sodium diet. In diuretic-resistant ascites, shunting may be performed in a number of ways:

- Peritoneovenous shunting (Le Veen shunt), where a subcutaneous silastic catheter is used to drain the fluid into the jugular vein
- The Denver shunt is a modification, adding a small subcutaneous pump that can be compressed externally
- Transjugular intrahepatic portosystemic stent shunt (TIPS), a side-to-side shunt stenting a channel between a branch of the portal vein and the hepatic vein

Note that interventional radiology techniques have largely replaced the surgically difficult open techniques.

FURTHER READING

Yu A S, Hu K Q (2001) Management of ascites. *Clin Liver Dis* **5**(2): 541–68, viii.
Suzuki H, Stanley A J (2001) Current management and novel therapeutic strategies for refractory ascites and hepatorenal syndrome. *QJM* **94**(6): 293–300.

** EPIGASTRIC MASS   CASE 58

INSTRUCTION

'Examine this lady's abdomen.'

APPROACH

Expose the patient and begin, as in Case 43, with the hands.

VITAL POINTS

Inspect peripheral signs

- Look for signs of anaemia in the hands and eyes
- Look for evidence of jaundice
- Palpate the supraclavicular fossa for lymphadenopathy (especially for a Virchow's node in the left supraclavicular fossa)

Inspect abdominal signs

- Comment on the presence of any scars
- There may be epigastric fullness

Palpate

Begin palpating as in Case 43, but stop when you find the mass and describe the mass fully before moving on. Comment on the:

- Size
- Surface
- Edge
- Consistency
- Relations – to the skin, to the costal margin, to the abdominal muscles
- Could the mass be hepatomegaly or splenomegaly?

Finish your examination here
Completion

Tell the examiner that you would carry on to complete the rest of the abdominal examination.

QUESTIONS

(a) What is the differential diagnosis?

As with right iliac fossa masses (*see* Case 55), the best way to think about this answer is to consider the possible diagnoses anatomically. You are less likely to forget any of the potential answers.

Arising from the skin and soft tissues:
- Sebaceous cysts
- Sarcoma

- Lipoma
- Hernia (epigastric)

Arising from the gastrointestinal tract:
- Hepatomegaly
- Carcinoma of the stomach
- Carcinoma of the pancreas (remember Courvoisier's Law – a palpable gallbladder in the presence of obstructive jaundice is not likely to be due to gallstones)
- Pancreatic pseudocyst

Arising from the vascular system:
- Abdominal aortic aneurysm (*see* Case 115)
- Retroperitoneal lymphadenopathy

Ludwig Georg Courvoisier (1843–1918). Professor of Surgery, Basle, Switzerland.

CASE 59   PLEURAL EFFUSION   ★★

INSTRUCTION

'Examine this gentleman's chest.'

APPROACH

Expose the patient from the waist up and sit him at 45° on the bed. Begin by examining the hands for peripheral stigmata of chronic respiratory disease.

VITAL POINTS

Inspect

In the hands and wrists, look for:

- Digital clubbing
- Nicotine (tar) staining of the fingers
- Pale palmar skin creases secondary to anaemia
- Hypertrophic pulmonary osteoarthropathy

In the neck, note the:

- Position of the jugular venous pulse
- Presence of supraclavicular lymphadenopathy
- Whether the trachea is central

Inspect the chest wall for:

- Scars
- Abdominal breathing

Note the respiratory rate while you are completing the peripheral examination (may be breathless with a large effusion).

Palpate

- Check expansion of the chest wall, noting whether it is equal bilaterally

Percuss

- Percuss the chest wall from the upper zone down, comparing the percussion note on both sides
- Repeat the process on the posterior chest wall (where effusions will be easier to hear)
- The percussion note is 'stony dull' on the side of the effusion

Auscultate

- Auscultate using the bell over the apices and the diaphragm elsewhere
- Diminished breath sounds will be heard over the effusion
- Vocal resonance will also be reduced
- Bronchial breathing may be heard if there is associated consolidation of the lung parenchyma

Finish your examination here

Completion

Tell the examiner you would:

- Examine the sputum pot
- Check the temperature
- Examine for potential causes of a pleural effusion (see below)

QUESTIONS

(a) How may pleural effusions be classified?

The protein content of a sample of effusion fluid is measured and the classification depends on this value:

- Transudate = protein < 30 g/l
- Exudate = protein > 30 g/l

(b) What are the causes of a pleural effusion?

See Table 17.

Table 17

Transudate	Exudate

Cardiac failure
Medical disorders leading
   to hypoalbuminaemia:
• Cirrhosis
• Nephrotic syndrome
	Malignancy
	• Primary lung tumour
	• Secondary (especially breast, GI, ovary)
	• Lymphoma
	• Chylothorax secondary
	      to malignant infiltration
	      of lymph
	Cardiovascular:
	• Pulmonary embolus/infarct
	• Dressler's syndrome (post myocardial infarct)
	Infections:
	• Pneumonia
	• Tuberculosis
	• Subphrenic abscess
	Systemic diseases:
	• Rheumatoid arthritis
	• Systemic lupus erythematosis

ADVANCED QUESTIONS

(a) How would you diagnose and treat a pleural effusion?

When the diagnosis has been made and confirmed with a plain film of the chest, a sample should be taken for:

• Biochemistry (including protein)
• Microbiology
• Cytology

Pleural taps are most easily performed in the mid-scapular line with the patient leaning forward over a table. Closed-needle biopsy of the pleura can also be performed – combined with cytology, this will diagnose 90% of malignancies and 75% cases of tuberculosis.

Treatment:

• If the patient remains symptomatic the fluid should be drained with a 14 gauge cannula
• Occasionally the pleural space may be obliterated using talc powder

(b) Under what situations would a chest drain be required to manage a pleural effusion?

Exudates that recur after aspiration require drainage and they may be placed on low suction (2.5–5 kPa); unlike drainage of a pneumothorax, these drains may be interrupted periodically to allow mobilization. The drain is left until the volume of fluid is < 100 ml/day and there is radiological re-expansion of the lung

> William Dressler (1890–1969). Cardiologist, Maimonides Hospital, New York.
> He described fever, chest pain, pericardial and pleural rub developing 2–10
> weeks after a myocardial infarction. It is thought to be due to an antibody
> reaction to heart muscle.

FURTHER READING

Peak G J, Morcos S, Cooper G (2000) The pleural cavity. *BMJ* **320**: 1318–21.
Ferrer J, Roldan J (2000) Investigation of pleural effusion. *Eur J Radiol* **34**(2):
76–86.

www.pulmonologychannel.com/pleuraleffusion – US site for respiratory
physicians.

** DYSPHAGIA   CASE 60

INSTRUCTION

'Ask this lady a few questions about her swallowing.'

APPROACH

It is useful to group your questions in terms of aetiologies and to let the examiner
know you are conscious of the possible more serious pathologies.

VITAL POINTS

- Are you having difficulty swallowing liquids, or solids, or both?
- Did the problem start suddenly or was the onset gradual?
- Do you ever regurgitate food?
- Can you eat a full meal?
- How long have you had this problem for?
- Where does the food stick – in the back of the throat, bottom of the neck or
  bottom of the chest?
- Do you ever get any pain – when you swallow or at other times?
- Have you had any weight-loss?
- Have you had a chest infection recently?

QUESTIONS

(a) What are the causes of dysphagia?

See Table 18.

Table 18   Causes of dysphagia

Mechanical obstruction	Co-ordination abnormalities

Within the lumen:
• Foreign body
• Oesophageal web
  (e.g. in scleroderma)
• Plummer–Vinson syndrome
  (Paterson–Brown–Kelly syndrome)
In the wall:
• Carcinoma of the oesophagus
• Oesophagitis (due to burns or
  chronic reflux)
• Barrett's oesophagus
• Benign oesophageal stricture
• Post-radiation strictures
Outside the wall:
• Retrosternal goitre
• Lung carcinoma
• Pharyngeal pouch
	Motility disorders:
	• Diffuse oesophageal spasm
	• Achalasia
	Neurological disease:
	• Myaesthenia gravis
	• Bulbar palsy including motor
	  neurone disease
	• Cerebrovascular accident
	  (with involvement of the 9th, 10th
	  or 12th cranial nerves or a
	  coordination difficulty)

(b) Which of these conditions are premalignant?

• Barrett's oesophagus
• Strictures secondary to radiation
• Achalasia
• Plummer–Vinson syndrome

(c) How do carcinomas of the oesophagus present?

• The characteristic presentation is insidious with progressive weight-loss and dysphagia
• The patient initially has difficulty swallowing solids and often describes the food getting stuck in the lower part of the oesophagus
• They may also describe odynophagia – pain on swallowing
• Occasionally they present with aspiration pneumonia

(d) What other conditions cause odynophagia?

• Infections within the oesophagus (especially candidiasis, herpes simplex)
• Pharyngitis
• Occasionally ulceration over the lower third of the oesophagus

ADVANCED QUESTIONS

(a) Which radiological investigations would you use in a patient whom you thought might be suffering from a dysmotility problem?

A barium swallow is the most useful test:

- In diffuse oesophageal spasm, a motor disorder of smooth muscle, below the aortic arch, normal coordinated peristalsis is replaced by multiple spontaneous contractions and this gives the characteristic 'corkscrew' oesophagus appearance
- Achalasia is a motility disorder due to loss of ganglia in the myenteric plexus, causing incomplete relaxation of the lower oesophageal sphincter; the oesophagus has a 'rats tail' appearance on the barium swallow and there is no gas bubble in the stomach

Endoscopy:

- If the diagnosis is in doubt, endoscopy with biopsies and brushings should be performed to exclude a carcinoma

---

D. R. Paterson (1863–1939). ENT surgeon at the Cardiff Royal Infirmary, described the association of glossitis, anaemia and dysphagia.
A. Brown-Kelly (1865–1941). British ENT surgeon; also described congenital stenosis as well as problems with motility.
H. S. Plummer (1874–1936). US physician working at the Mayo clinic, who investigated the therapeutic use of oxygen in respiratory disease, and was interested in the diagnostic and therapeutic use of bronchoscopy and endoscopy.
P. P. Vinson (1890–1959). US physician also working at the Mayo clinic.

FURTHER READING

Owen W (2001) Dysphagia. *BMJ* **323**: 850–3.

www.healthinfocus.co.uk/ – explains the different types of gastrooesophageal reflux disease, with links to descriptions of the causes.

CASE 61   ENLARGED KIDNEY   **

INSTRUCTION

'Examine this gentleman's abdomen.'

APPROACH

Expose the patient and begin with the hand (Case 43).

VITAL POINTS

Inspect

- Inspection is likely to be normal

Palpate

- In advanced renal tumours, there may be supraclavicular lymphadenopathy
- Note the presence of a mass in the left or right loins or upper quadrants
- This mass must be distinguished from other causes of masses:
  - an enlarged kidney descends with inspiration as it is pushed down by the diaphragm
  - it can be balloted (bimanual palpation with the right hand behind the left side of the patient's abdomen pushing upwards, feeling the kidney with the left hand held on the abdominal wall at the front)
  - the hand can get in between the swelling and the costal margin
  - the percussion note is nearly always resonant because there is colon between the skin and the kidney

Finish your examination here

QUESTIONS

(a) What is the differential diagnosis for an enlarged kidney?

Congenital:

- Cystic disease (including polycystic kidney disease)
- Horseshoe kidney
- Hypertrophic single kidney

Acquired:

- Diseases specific to the kidney:
  - solitary cysts
  - tumours
  - hydronephrosis
  - pyonephrosis
  - perinephric abscess
  - renal vein thrombosis

- As part of systemic disease:
  - diabetes
  - amyloidosis
  - systemic lupus erythematosis

(b) What are the differences between infantile and adult polycystic kidney disease?

See Table 19.

Table 19 Polycystic kidney disease

	Adult	**Infantile**
Inheritance	Autosomal dominant	Autosomal recessive
Incidence	1 in 500	1 in 5000–40 000
Genetics	Chromosomes 4,16	6
Age of presentation	30s–50s	Perinatal
Pattern of presentation	Hypertension	Oligohydramnios
	Haematuria	Large liver and kidneys
	Loin pain	Chronic renal failure
Pattern of enlargement	Asymmetrical	Symmetrical
Liver involvement	Adult liver cysts common	Always congenital hepatic fibrosis
		Sometimes biliary ectasia
Other systemic involvement	Intracranial aneurysms	None
	Colonic diverticulae	
	Mitral regurgitation	
Prognosis	Often require dialysis but good prognosis	All die by age 20, but often in neonatal period

(c) What is the normal mode of presentation of renal cell carcinomas?

- Usually occur in the over 50s
- Classic presentation is a triad (Beck's triad) of:
  - haematuria
  - mass
  - loin pain
- Other presentations:
  - incidentally found on abdominal ultrasound or CT scans performed for another reason (very common)
  - pyrexia of unknown origin
  - anaemia of chronic disease
  - polycythaemia (due to erythropoietin secretion by the tumour)
  - raised erythrocyte sedimentation rate
  - hypercalcaemia
  - left-sided varicocele

ADVANCED QUESTIONS

(a) Simple cysts are found in 33% of patients by the age of 60. How should they be managed?

History and clinical examination:

- They usually present incidentally but occasionally with a renal mass or haematuria

Investigations:

- Blood tests would be expected to be normal
- A renal ultrasound scan shows a cyst with a smooth outline, sharply defined thin wall and no internal echoes (which imply solid components)

Treatment:

- The major differential diagnoses would be with a renal tumour and adult polycystic kidney disease and if there is any doubt of a tumour, then the cyst fluid may be sent for cytological analysis

(b) What radiological features would make you suspicious of an occult renal cell carcinoma?

More worrying features for a tumour would include:

- Thick, or irregular wall
- Extensive calcification within the cavity or wall of the cyst
- Multilocular cysts

FURTHER READING

Tomson C R (2000) Recent advances: nephrology. *BMJ* **320**(7227): 98–101.
Godley P A, Taylor M (2001) Renal cell carcinoma. *Curr Opin Oncol* **13**(3): 199–203.

www.pkdcure.org – website of the polycystic foundation, a worldwide organization devoted to determining the cause and treatment for polycystic kidney disease.

* COMMON SURGICAL SCARS | CASE 62

INSTRUCTION

'Inspect this gentleman's abdomen.'

APPROACH

Introduce yourself and expose the patient's abdomen, positioning him flat on the bed. Leave his external genitalia covered at this point to maintain his dignity but expose the whole of the top half of his body down to the symphysis pubis. If the examiner indicates the patient should leave his shirt on, then expose from above the xiphisternum to the symphysis pubis.

VITAL POINTS

Inspect

Comment on the presence of any surgical scars (Fig. 23):

- Use the correct technical names for the scars where possible, if not describe the anatomical position of the scar and indicate whether it looks well healed or recently formed
- You should not guess at the operation the patient underwent in order to produce the scar unless asked specifically to do so by the examiner

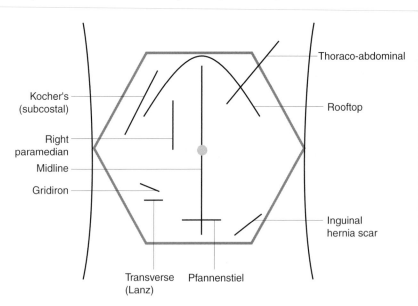

Fig. 23 Common surgical scars. Remember to examine the flanks for the loin incision of a nephrectomy.

> **TOP TIP**
> When you see a scar on the abdomen, always think of the presence of an incisional hernia (*see* Case 47). From the end of the bed, ask the patient to raise their head off the bed and cough in order to demonstrate this. Continue to examine each scar more carefully during the Palpation section to rule out incisional herniae.

Finish your examination here

QUESTIONS

(a) Which operation do you think this patient may have had?

Although you should not make guesses at which operation a particular patient may have had in order to produce the named scar, in the short cases and OSCEs the examiner may ask you for an educated opinion.

There may be a few pointers:

- Is there evidence of a new or old stoma site (from a bowel operation)?
- Is there evidence of a small incision to one side of the scar (from a drain – this may have been due to a bowel operation)?
- Are there also scars in the groins (perhaps ilio-femoral segment surgery in a patient who has also had an abdominal aortic aneurysm repaired through a midline incision)?
- Are there striae gravidarum (Pfannenstiel incision may have been for a Caesarean section)?

> *Herman Johannes Pfannensteil (1862–1909).* Gynaecologist from Breslau who described the popular curved suprapubic incision.

CASE 63   BREAST EXAMINATION –   *
GENERAL APPROACH

INSTRUCTION

'Examine this lady's breast.'

APPROACH

Before beginning this examination, whether in a long case or short case, you must be accompanied by a chaperone, and a nurse will be available for this purpose in the examination.

Expose the patient from the waist up and lie her at 45° on the couch.

VITAL POINTS

Inspect

Begin by asking the patient if they have noticed a lump in the breast, and which breast this is in.

Stand away from the couch and look at the patient's breasts from the front

- Ask the patient to lift both her hands above her head, stretching the skin and emphasizing any tethering of a breast tumour to the skin
- Next, ask her to place both her hands on her hips, and while watching her breasts, ask her to press firmly into the hips with both hands; this emphasizes any attachment of a breast tumour to the underlying pectoralis major muscle, which contracts with this manoeuvre

Move closer to the patient and look more closely at the breasts:

- Inspect the nipple and areola (*see* Top Tip)
- Inspect the rest of the breasts for:
  - asymmetry in size or shape
  - skin changes or subcutaneous nodules
  - previous scars from excision of benign or malignant lumps

---

TOP TIP – THE SEVEN 'D'S OF NIPPLE SIGNS
When inspecting the nipple, or taking a history of nipple symptoms:

- Discolouration
- Discharge
- Depression (often referred to as inversion)
- Deviation
- Displacement
- Destruction
- (Duplication – unlikely in the exam)

Palpate

Ask the patient to tell you where the lump in the breast is first, but start by palpating the normal breast. When examining the left breast, ask the patient to place her left hand behind her neck, stretching the left breast over the thoracic wall:

- Palpate systemically round the breast, using the tips of your fingers held together
- Retract the breast with the left hand and use the right hand to palpate each of the four quadrants
- Imagine the breast as a clock face and make sure that each area is palpated
- Pay particular attention to the axillary tail and underneath the nipple where masses are frequently missed
- When palpating the abnormal breast, ensure that the area of abnormality that you have found is the same that the patient has noticed
- The location of the lump within the breast should be named according to the quadrant (upper outer, lower outer, upper inner, lower inner)

- Describe any lump as in Case 1, noting whether it is attached to the skin or the underlying muscle
- Palpate the five areas of lymph nodes in the axilla – medial, lateral, anterior, posterior and apical (Fig. 24) – palpating the left axilla with your right hand and vice versa
- Palpate the supraclavicular fossa for lymphadenopathy and apical) (Fig. 24), palpating.

Finish your examination here

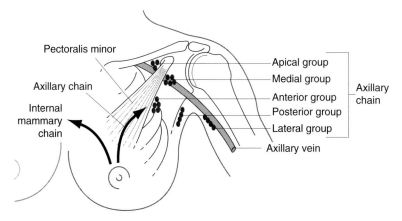

Fig. 24   Lymph nodes and lymphatic drainage of the breast.

Completion

Tell the examiner you would continue by:
- Percussing and auscultating the chest
- Palpating the abdomen for hepatomegaly
- Percussing the axial spine for tenderness
- Complete a general physical examination to determine the patient's fitness for surgery

FURTHER READING

www.cancernet.nci.nih.gov/Understanding/ABTLUMPS.html – website from the US describing different types of breast lump with information about the pathogenesis of each.

http://www.infobreastcancer.cyberus.ca/bse2.htm – a pictorial guide to breast self-examination for women.

* BREAST LUMP   CASE 64

INSTRUCTION

'Examine this lady's breasts.'

APPROACH

Expose the patient to the waist to adequately expose the breasts and chest wall.

VITAL POINTS

Inspect

- The lump may be tethered to the skin or underlying muscle
- There may be associated nipple changes, or changes to the skin of the breast
- There may be scars from previous surgery

Palpate

As in Case 63, begin with the normal breast, examining with the patient's hand behind her head. When you have identified the lump, describe the lump in detail:

- Site (position) – name the quadrant the lump is located within
- Size – measure the lump approximately
- Surface – smooth/irregular/nodular
- Edge – well/poorly defined
- Consistency – soft/firm/hard
- Tenderness
- Fluctuation
- Fixation – to skin or the underlying chest wall

Continue as in Case 63 by palpating the axilla and supraclavicular fossa and complete the examination as in Case 63.

Finish your examination here

QUESTIONS

(a) How would you investigate this patient?

The buzzword here is TRIPLE ASSESSMENT, which consists of:

- History and physical examination
- Imaging (ultrasound or mammography)
- Cytology (fine-needle aspiration or occasionally a Trucut biopsy)

(b) What is the differential diagnosis of a breast lump?

Single lumps in the breast are most likely to be:

- Fibroadenomas
- Breast cysts
- Breast cancer

(c) What features of the lump would make you suspicious that it is a breast cancer?

- Surface – irregular or nodular
- Edge – poorly defined, with areas which are more like normal breast tissue in between more abnormal areas
- Consistency – breast tumours are usually firm, rather than hard
- Tenderness – usually non-tender
- Fluctuation – usually not fluctuant
- Fixation – to skin or the underlying chest wall
- Any involvement of the nipple in the lump or concurrent nipple changes

Also mention the presence of any lymphadenopathy, or features in the history or physical examination, that suggest disseminated disease.

(d) What are the characteristic clinical features of fibroadenomas and breast cysts?

Fibroadenomas:

- Benign tumours developing from a single breast lobule
- Hormonally dependent – involute after the menopause and increase in size with menstruation
- Commonly present in women between 15 and 25 years old
- Well defined, regular, smooth, firm mass
- Freely mobile within the breast ('breast mouse')

Breast cysts:

- Distended, involuted lobules
- Most common in women between 40 and 55 years old (perimenopausal)
- Usually fluctuant
- Can be painful
- Well defined and smooth
- Can be multiple

FURTHER READING

Houssami N, Cheung M N, Dixon J M (2001) Fibroadenoma of the breast. *Med J Aust* **174**(4): 185–8.

Drukker B H (1994) Fibrocystic change of the breast. *Clin Obstet Gynecol* **37**(4): 903–15.

www.medstat.med.utah.edu/webpath/TUTORIAL/BREAST/BREAST.html – tutorial on differential diagnosis of breast lumps.

* POST-MASTECTOMY BREAST CASE 65

INSTRUCTION

'Examine this lady's breasts.'

APPROACH

Expose the patient and begin examining the breasts as in Case 63.

VITAL POINTS

Inspect

- Note the asymmetrical chest wall and describe the location of the scar
- Look at the surrounding skin and into the axilla determining whether there has also been radiotherapy to the surrounding area
- Ask the patient to press her hands into her hips, ascertaining whether the pectoralis major remains underneath the mastectomy

Palpate

- It is likely that you would not have to continue to palpate the breast, but if the examiner wants you to continue, you should examine the remaining breast as in Case 63
- Palpate the axilla and supraclavicular fossa for lymphadenopathy

Finish your examination here

Completion

Tell the examiner you would examine the abdomen, neck, lung fields and spine. You would also examine the ipsilateral arm for lymphoedema.

QUESTIONS

(a) What are the indications for mastectomy?

Modern breast surgery has tended to become more conservative, and no survival benefit has ever been demonstrated in performing more radical breast surgery for isolated breast carcinomas.

There are some occasions where mastectomy is indicated:

- Large lumps (depends on the size of the breast but often defined as > 4 cm)
- Involvement of the nipple
- Multifocal carcinomas
- Ductal carcinoma *in situ*

ADVANCED QUESTIONS

(a) What different types of mastectomy can be performed?

- SIMPLE MASTECTOMY – removal of the breast alone

The following procedures are rarely performed now as survival benefit has not been demonstrated:

- MODIFIED RADICAL MASTECTOMY (Patey) – removal of the breast, pectoralis minor and the axillary structures
- RADICAL MASTECTOMY (Halsted mastectomy) – removal of the breast, pectoralis major and minor, and the axillary contents
- EXTENDED RADICAL MASTECTOMY – as for the radical procedure but also removing the internal mammary nodes (between the 2nd and 4th anterior intercostal spaces)

The disadvantage with simple mastectomy, although least disfiguring, is that the axilla still needs to be managed following surgery (for instance with radiotherapy), whereas the other types involve surgical dissection of the axillary nodes. Postoperative radiotherapy is more common for limited resections.

(b) How would you prepare a patient prior to mastectomy?

Physical preparation:

- Mark the side prior to anaesthetic
- Explanation of the procedure should include the use of a suction drain to close the cavity following surgery and decrease the risk of scar and haematoma formation
- An anaesthetized patch of skin in the axilla and the upper medial part of the arm will follow division of the intercostobrachial nerve (T1), which is divided as it emerges from the chest wall just posterior to the origin of the pectoralis minor muscle
- Anaesthetic workup should include chest X-ray to exclude pulmonary metastasis

Psychological preparation:

- All patients should see the breast care nurse preoperatively and the reasons for mastectomy should be discussed fully
- The option of reconstructive surgery (*see* Case 66) should be discussed

(c) When should the drains be removed post-surgery?

- Often surgeons place two drains, one in the axilla and one lower down in the cavity
- The drains are usually left for 3–5 days, or until the drainage volume is < 50 ml in one day
- Patients can safely be sent home with drains in place and district nurse support, as otherwise they may spend a week in hospital

> *William Stewart Halsted (1852–1922).* First Professor of Surgery at Johns Hopkins Medical School, Baltimore, where Harvey Cushing was his assistant. He also introduced rubber gloves to surgery (made for him by the company Goodyear) and was one of the first to use regional anaesthesia with cocaine.

FURTHER READING

Eatock J (2000) Counselling in primary care: past, present and future. *Br J Guidance & Counselling* **28**(2): 161–73.

www.cancerweb.ncl.ac.uk/cancernet/ – patient-focused website with details of the procedure and expectations following mastectomy.

---

* **BREAST RECONSTRUCTION**   **CASE 66**

INSTRUCTION

'Examine this lady's chest wall.'

APPROACH

Expose the patient as in Case 63.

VITAL POINTS

Inspect

- Note the asymmetry of the chest wall
- The prosthesis can be identified by the presence of surgical scars and by a different shape from the normal breast contour

Flap reconstruction

- More extensive surgical scarring
- Scars extend over the back or abdominal wall
- Look at the patient's back and see the recess where the latissimus dorsi has been removed
- Ask the patient to lift their head off the bed (when lying flat) to see the recess in the rectus abdominis muscle

Implant reconstruction

- Shape is rounder than a 'normal' breast
- Lie of the breast is usually higher
- A Becker implant may have a palpable subcutaneous filling port in the axilla

Finish your examination here

> TOP TIP
> Do not be embarrassed to ask the patient for permission to examine the reconstructed breast and the other breast. Do so with confidence. In this situation it is useful to inform the examiner of your findings on inspection prior to palpation.

ADVANCED QUESTIONS

(a) What are the possible types of breast reconstruction surgery?

- Subcutaneous prosthesis
- Submuscular implant
- Tissue expander
- Myocutaneous flap
  - transverse rectus abdominis myocutaneous (TRAM) flap
  - latissimus dorsi (LD flap)

(b) What are the advantages and disadvantages of using an implant?

See Table 20.

Table 20   Using an implant

Advantages	Disadvantages
Technique simpler than flaps	Cosmetic result less satisfactory than using a flap
Place under the pectoralis muscles to reduce the incidence of contraction of the capsule	Requires plenty of available skin following surgery
Can be performed at the time of the mastectomy or at a later date	Lies above the natural inframammary fold, leaving the breast higher than the other one

(c) What are the advantages and disadvantages of myocutaneous flaps?

See Table 21.

Table 21   Myocutaneous flaps

Advantages	Disadvantages
Useful where remaining skin and muscle in short supply, e.g. following extensive surgery	May need to be performed in combination with plastic surgeon
	Greater blood loss
Cosmetic results can be very good	Greater operating time and operative complications
Suitable for use post-mastectomy	Use of rectus abdominus may be impossible if the patient has had previous abdominal surgery
Suitable for salvage after local recurrence	Late complications include flap necrosis and infection

FURTHER READING

Malyon A D, Husein M, Weiler-Mithoff E M (2001) How many procedures to make a breast? *Br J Plast Surg* **54**(3): 227–31.

Malata C M, McIntosh S A, Purushotham A D (2000) Immediate breast reconstruction after mastectomy for cancer. *Br J Surg* **87**(11): 1455–72.

www.cancerbacup.org.uk/info/breast-reconstruction.html – booklet written by women who have undergone breast reconstruction surgery and reviewed by editorial panel including oncologists and specialist nurses.

www.fda.gov/cdrh/ – centres for devices which explains different types of prostheses that are licensed in the US and the pros and cons of each (also has all other types of medical and surgical prostheses).

* GYNAECOMASTIA CASE 67

INSTRUCTION

'Look at this gentleman's chest.'

APPROACH

Expose the patient as for the chest examination and position him at 45°.

VITAL POINTS

Inspect

Note the presence of unilateral or bilateral breast swellings. They may be simply small breast buds, or more significant amounts of breast tissue may be present.

Finish your examination here

Completion

Tell the examiner you would look for a cause of the gynaecomastia, including examination of the external genitalia, examining for clinical signs of thyroid dysfunction, and for signs of liver disease. You would ask the patient some directed questions, especially about the use of prescription or recreational drugs.

QUESTIONS

(a) What are the causes of gynaecomastia?

Physiological:

- Particularly common at puberty where the patient may have noticed unilateral or bilateral gynaecomastia – may enlarge to considerable size but usually disappear before adulthood

Drugs:

- Recreational drugs: marijuana, amphetamines, diazepam
- Gastrointestinal drugs: cimetidine, ranitidine
- Cardiovascular drugs: digoxin, angiotensin converting enzyme inhibitors (e.g. captopril, enalapril), spironolactone, nifedipine, verapamil
- Antibiotics: metronidazole, isoniazid, ketoconazole

Endocrine disorders:

- Hypo or hyperthyroidism
- Hypogonadism, in testicular atrophy, and Klinefelter's syndrome
- Acromegaly

Malignancy:

- Testicular tumours
- Lymphoma

Liver disease:

- Usually alcoholic cirrhosis

ADVANCED QUESTIONS

(a) How might you investigate this patient?

The level of investigation depends very much on the clinical situation, and some patients may require no investigations at all. Possible useful investigations would include:

- Plasma alpha feto-protein and beta-human chorionic gonadotrophin – raised levels may indicate a testicular tumour
- Testosterone and luteinizing hormone levels to demonstrate hypogonadism
- Thyroid function tests

(b) What would make you concerned the patient may have a breast cancer?

Male breast cancer is responsible for 1% of all cases of breast cancer in the UK. Features that would be suspicious include:

- Older age
- Unilateral gynaecomastia
- Firm or hard nodules within the breast tissue (the texture is normally rubbery or soft)
- Remember to examine the axillary and supraclavicular fossae for lymphadenopathy

If in doubt, the patient should undergo triple assessment (*see* Case 64) including imaging and fine-needle aspirate cytology.

Harry Fitch Klinefelter Jr (born 1912). Associate Professor of Medicine at Johns Hopkins University – the syndrome in its full form is known as Klinefelter-Reifenstein-Albright syndrome.
Fuller Albright (1900–1969). Professor of Medicine, Harvard Medical School who contributed a huge amount to the study of metabolic diseases.
E.C. Reifenstein also worked with Albright. Reifenstein syndrome is male pseudohermaphroditism.

FURTHER READING

Neuman J F (1997) Evaluation and treatment of gynecomastia. *Am Fam Physician* 55(5): 1835–44, 1849–50.
www.abc.net.ac/rn/talks/8.30/helthrpt/stories/s300553.htm – transcript of a radio interview given in May 2001 on Australian radio discussing the presentation and treatment of gynaecomastia (with a UK specialist)

POST LOBECTOMY/PNEUMONECTOMY CHEST CASE 68

INSTRUCTION

'Examine this gentleman's chest.'

APPROACH

Position the patient and begin to examine the chest as in Case 59, beginning with the hands, but expect that the examiner may move you directly on to examining the chest wall

VITAL POINTS

Inspect

- Note the lateral thoracotomy scar over the chest wall – the scar begins at the sternal end of the 5th or 6th intercostal space and curves posteriorly and upwards, ending midway between the spine of the scapula and the thoracic vertebral spines.
- Scars at the sites of chest drains may be present
- Muscle bulk over the side of the scar may be reduced as parts of serratus anterior and latissimus dorsi may have been removed

Palpate

- The trachea is deviated away from the side of surgery
- Expansion will be reduced over the side of surgery

Percuss

- Percussion note over the side of surgery is hyper-resonant

Auscultate

- Breath sounds are harsher over the side of the pneumonectomy

Finish your examination here

QUESTIONS

(a) What are the indications for lung resections?

- 90% of lung resections in the Western world are performed for bronchial carcinoma
- Other indications include:
  - bronchiectasis
  - chronic infection including tuberculosis
  - benign tumours (e.g. carcinoid)
  - metastatic tumours

(b) What are the types of lung resection?

- Lobectomy is the excision of a single lobe of the lung
- Pneumonectomy is the excision of an entire lung
- Sleeve resection is the resection of a lobe including its bronchial origin with re-anastamosis of the proximal and distal bronchus

ADVANCED QUESTIONS

(a) What is the operative mortality for lung resections?

A recent retrospective study looked at 442 patients who had undergone lobectomy and pneumonectomy over an 18-year period (see Further Reading). The operative mortality for lobectomy was 7% and for pneumonectomy 12%, but no difference in long-term survival was detected. Techniques such as sleeve lobectomy and bronchoplasty have been developed as a result of the high operative mortality of pneumonectomy. Risk of operative mortality is higher with:

- Higher American Society of Anaesthesiologists score (preoperative morbidity)
- Age > 70 years
- Poor respiratory function especially FEV_1/FVC ratio of < 55%

FURTHER READING

Ferguson M K, Karrison T (2000) Does pneumonectomy for lung cancer adversely influence long-term survival? *J Thorac Cardiovasc Surg* **119**(3): 440–8.

Groenendijk R P, Croiset van Uchelen F A, Mol S J, de Munck D R, Tan A T, Roumen R M (1999) Factors related to outcome after pneumonectomy: retrospective study of 62 patients. *Eur J Surg* **165**(3): 193–7.

INSTRUCTION

'Examine this gentleman's chest.'

APPROACH

Expose the patient to examine the chest as in Case 59.

VITAL POINTS

Inspect

- The median sternotomy scar runs from the suprasternal notch vertically in the midline to the xiphisternum
- Subtotal median sternotomy involves an incision from the sternomanubrial junction to the 5th or 6th intercostal space

Palpate

- Occasionally there is non-union of the two sides of the manubrium sternum when a 'click' can be felt on palpation
- Unless there is co-morbidity, the examiner wants you to pick up that the rest of the thoracic examination is likely to be normal

Finish your examination here

QUESTIONS

(a) What are the indications for median sternotomy?

- Emergency procedures, e.g. following penetrating chest trauma
- Cardiac surgery
- Resection of lung cancer

There is some evidence that median sternotomy may be as efficient an approach to the lung as the lateral thoracotomy (see Further Reading)

ADVANCED QUESTIONS

(a) What are the principles of cardiopulmonary bypass?

- The aim of bypass is to provide a systemic circulation while the heart is stopped and emptied of blood (Fig. 25)
- Blood is drained by gravity from the right heart to a circuit where, after gas and temperature exchange, it is returned to the arterial side of the circulation

- The components of the perfusion circuit are:
  - an oxygenator – oxygen added and carbon dioxide removed from the blood
  - a heat exchanger – initially blood is cooled, later in the procedure it is warmed again
  - cardiotomy suction – pericardial sump suckers return spilt blood to the circulation
  - roller pump – returns blood to the aorta
  - arterial line filter – removes debris and matter from the circulation

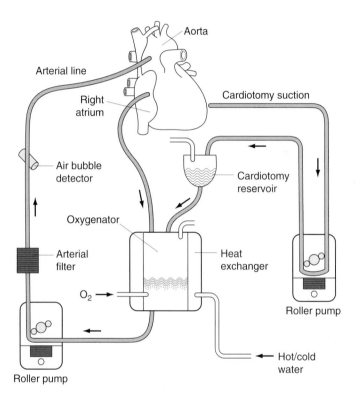

Fig. 25 Components of a cardiopulmonary bypass circuit.

(b) What are the major complications of bypass?

- Systemic activation of inflammatory mediators causes coagulopathy
- Cerebral damage due to ischaemia (1–2%)
- Microemboli, e.g. to kidneys, terminal arteries in limbs, retina

FURTHER READING

Asaph J W, Handy J R Jr, Grunkemeier G L, *et al.* (2000) Median sternotomy versus thoracotomy to resect primary lung cancer: analysis of 815 cases. *Ann Thorac Surg* **70**(2): 373–9.

INSTRUCTION

'Examine this gentleman's scrotum.'

APPROACH

See Case 51.

VITAL POINTS

Inspect

The scrotum may look normal but often an enlarged testis is visible

Palpate

The mass is:

- Usually inseparable from the testis
- Hard, irregular, nodular
- Non tender
- Not transilluminable
- Distinct from the superficial inguinal ring (you can 'get above' the mass)

It may have an associated hydrocele and there may be some thickening of the spermatic cord due to malignant infiltration.

Finish your examination here

Completion

Always remember to examine the contralateral scrotum. Tell the examiner you would continue to examine for abdominal lymphadenopathy, and you would perform an examination of the abdomen (for hepatomegaly) and chest (for thoracic metastates).

QUESTIONS

(a) What is the differential diagnosis?

- Testicular tumours can be mimicked by chronic or old infection leading to scarring, such as in orchitis or tuberculosis
- Occasionally a long-standing hydrocele may develop calcification and become harder, clinically similar to a tumour
- Tumours occasionally grow locally to become adherent to the inside of the scrotal skin, again it is possible for a chronic hydrocele to mimic this, but the level of suspicion of a tumour would be high

(b) How do testicular tumours usually present?

- The commonest presentation is a painless lump or a dull ache in one testis in a young man
- Occasionally there is a history of trauma accompanying the discovery of the mass
- 10% present with an acutely painful testis (which must be distinguished from a testicular torsion)
- If para-aortic nodes have become infiltrated with metastases, the patient may complain of back pain

(c) How is a testicular tumour removed?

Through an inguinal approach, with early clamping of the testicular artery and vein within the spermatic cord before the testis is mobilized out of the scrotum – this prevents intraoperative seeding of tumour up the testicular vein.

ADVANCED QUESTIONS

(a) What is the classification of testicular malignancies?

Almost all are seminomas or teratomas (see Table 22), other types are:

- Embryonal carcinoma (arising from a very primitive germ cell)
- Choriocarcinoma
- Yolk sac tumour
- Leydig cell tumours – associated with gynaecomastia, but only 10% are malignant
- Sertoli cell tumours – also produce gynaecomastia
- Lymphoma – most commonly in patients who have generalized lymphoma elsewhere and is generally associated with a poor prognosis

Table 22

	Teratoma	Seminoma
Age of presentation	20–30 years	30–40 years
Tumour markers	AFP and βHCG raised in 90%	Usually normal
Treatment of early disease	Chemotherapy (often only two cycles)	Radiotherapy to the para-aortic nodes +/– single dose of cisplatin
Treatment of advanced disease	Combination chemotherapy	Adjuvant chemotherapy, either single dose or in combination

Franz von Leydig (1821–1908). German histologist who first described the androgen-producing Leydig cell.
Enrico Sertoli (1842–1910). Professor of Experimental Physiology, Milan.

FURTHER READING

Dearnaley D, Huddart R, Horwich A (2001) Regular review: Managing testicular cancer. *BMJ* **322**(7302): 1583–8.

Oliver R T (2001) Testicular Cancer. *Curr Opin Oncol* **13**(3): 191–8.

www.icr.ac.uk/everyman/about/testicular.html – guide to testicular self-examination for patients

---

* ENTEROCUTANEOUS FISTULA   CASE 71

INSTRUCTION

'Inspect this gentleman's abdomen and comment on what you can see.'

APPROACH

Expose the patient as in Case 43 and inspect the abdominal wall; do not begin with the hands as you have been given a specific instruction to inspect the abdomen.

VITAL POINTS

Inspect

Describe the appearance of the fistula:

- Site
- Size
- Discharge (fluid/solid/colour) – material may be bile or faeces, etc.
- Surrounding skin (may be damaged by irradiation, inflammatory bowel disease or chemical irritation from small intestine contents)

Describe the rest of the abdominal wall:

- Presence of recent scar; an anastamotic leak may have led to the fistula
- Previous surgery – especially for malignancy or inflammatory bowel disease
- Presence of a stoma, healed stoma or drain sites

Comment on any other 'clues' around the bed:

- General condition of the patient (anaemic, cachectic, etc.)
- Drips and parenteral nutrition
- Catheters/central venous pressure lines

Finish your examination here

Completion

Tell the examiner you would examine the patient looking for an underlying aetiology (see below).

QUESTIONS

(a) What is the definition of an enterocutaneous fistula?

- A fistula is an abnormal connection between two epithelial or endothelial surfaces
- An enterocutaneous fistula is an abnormal connection between the gastrointestinal tract and the skin

(b) What is the aetiology of enterocutaneous fistulae?

Inflammation:

- Inflammatory bowel disease, especially Crohn's disease
- Diverticular disease
- Tuberculosis

Malignancy:

- Often following spontaneous rupture and abscess formation by the tumour

Radiotherapy:

- Pelvic irradiation can damage the intestine

Trauma:

- Penetrating wounds to the abdomen, especially involving the perforation of several separate loops of bowel with significant contamination and sepsis

Post-surgery:

- Anastamotic leak, often following primary anastamosis in contaminated conditions, e.g. sepsis or distal obstruction

ADVANCED QUESTIONS

(a) How may the anatomical locations of these fistulae be classified?

A high intestinal fistula involves the stomach, duodenum, jejunum and ileum and results in high volume fluid losses; a low fistula involves the large intestine and fluid losses are lower in volume.

(b) What investigations are required?

Blood tests:

- Full blood count – anaemia may be caused by haemorrhage and sepsis raises white cell count
- Blood cultures should be taken prior to commencement of antibiotics
- Electrolytes, especially to check the patient is not severely hypokalaemic
- Inflammatory markers (C-reactive protein, ESR)
- Liver function tests – reduced albumin indicates malnutrition

Radiological investigations:

- A fistulogram is the injection of contrast material into the fistula opening in order to see (using screening) where the fistula connects to the bowel
- This also allows for needle drainage of pockets of pus
- Ultrasound and CT scanning are used to determine the extent of the cavity and to detect underlying pathologies
- A barium follow-through or enema, depending on the site

(c) What are the principles of treatment?

- Early recourse to surgery (especially in high intestinal fistulae) carries extremely high risk
- These patients are nutritionally and fluid-depleted, losing litres of electrolyte-rich fluid through the fistula
- Management is similar to intestinal obstruction and involves careful fluid and electrolyte monitoring and intravenous fluid with added potassium and parenteral nutrition
- When the sepsis is controlled and distal obstruction has been relieved, 60% of fistulae should close spontaneously within 1 month

FURTHER READING

Metcalf C (1999) Enterocutaneous fistulae. *J Wound Care* **8**(3): 141–2.
Berry S M, Fischer J E (1996) Classification and pathophysiology of enterocutaneous fistulas. *Surg Clin North Am* **76**(5): 1009–18.

www.ibscrohns.about.com/library/weekly/aa071200a.htm – description of fistulae as applied to patients with Crohn's disease.

---

* MOUTH SIGNS IN ABDOMINAL DISEASE   CASE 72

INSTRUCTION

'Look inside this patient's mouth', or as part of 'Examine this gentleman's abdomen'.

VITAL POINTS

Inspect

Abnormalities within the mouth can be grouped according to the appearances seen.

Abnormal pigmentation

- Addison's disease – the mouth and lips are hyperpigmented
- Lichen planus – white lines and streaks inside the mouth
- Peutz–Jeghers disease – pigmented freckles around the lips and inside the mouth; associated with intestinal intussusception and gastrointestinal bleeding

from colonic polyps. The patients have a higher incidence of concurrent malignancy such as breast, lung and pancreatic carcinomas
- Hereditary telangiectasia (Rendu–Osler–Weber disease) – multiple telangiectasia (clusters of dilated capillaries and venules) around the mouth and on the tongue and lips; associated with gastrointestinal bleeding due to arteriovenous malformations; a group of clustered autosomal dominant conditions
- Acanthosis Nigricans – black discolouration of the skin, associated with carcinoma of the stomach and oesophagus, lymphomas and with endocrine disorders (acromegaly, Cushing's, diabetes complicated by severe insulin resistance)

Ulceration

- Aphthous ulcers are small, round and shallow, and have a shallow yellow base with surrounding erythema; they are common in childhood and are associated with infection and minor trauma to the oral cavity. In inflammatory bowel disease and coeliac disease, the ulcers tend to be more persistent and much larger; in Crohn's disease, the mouth takes on a 'cobblestone' appearance due to frequent ulceration, healing with some fibrosis
- Behcet's disease – a rare autoimmune disease most common in young men, causing a triad of genital and oral ulceration and anterior uveitis
- Herpes simplex – small vesicles with an erythematous base on the lips and inside of the mouth; diagnosed with scrapings of the base of the lesions and usually responsive to topical aciclovir

Lip disorders

- Angular stomatitis – chapping and splitting of the corners of the lips is normal, but can also occur in
  - herpes simplex and candidal infections
  - iron, folate, vitamin B and C deficiencies

Infections

- Herpes simplex causes both stomatitis and ulceration (above)
- Oral candidiasis is the most common abnormality; causes creamy white patches that may be rubbed off, and may be seen in:
  - patients prescribed inhaled steroids for the treatment of asthma and chronic obstructive airways disease (the patient information leaflet advises patients to wash their mouths out after using these inhalers)
  - oral antibiotic use
  - immunocompromised patients including those who are diabetic, and those on oral steroids

Henry Jules Louis Marie Rendu (1844–1902). Parisian physician.
Sir William Osler (1849–1919). Tremendously significant medical educator, who was Professor of Medicine at Johns Hopkins and Oxford Universities, and was responsible for the formation of the Association of Physicians of Great Britain and Northern Ireland, and for setting up full-time chairmen of medicine in London hospitals.
Frederick Parkes Weber (1863–1962). London physician.
Harvey Williams Cushing (1869–1939). 'The Founder of Neurosurgery' and Professor of Surgery, Harvard.
Halushi Behcet (1889–1948). Turkish dermatologist.
Thomas Addison (1793–1860). Physician at Guys hospital, who was by reputation an excellent diagnostician and lecturer. Known as the Founder of Endocrinology.
John Law Augustine Peutz (1886–1957). Dutch physician; Chief of Internal Medicine, St John's Hospital, The Hague.
Harald Jos Jeghers. Professor of Medicine, New Jersey College of Medicine and Dentistry, Jersey City.

---

* EPIGASTRIC HERNIA   CASE 73

INSTRUCTION

'Examine this gentleman's abdomen.'

APPROACH

Expose the patient and begin to examine as for Case 43.

VITAL POINTS

Inspect

- When asking the patient to lift his head off the bed, a lump may appear in the epigastric region, in the midline
- Ask him to cough and see if this lump becomes more prominent in the abdominal wall

Palpate

- Palpate the area of the hernia carefully
- It can be very difficult to find the hernia, ask the patient to help by again lifting the head off the bed and coughing
- Try to identify the borders of the defect and the size of the neck

---

TOP TIP

If there is no scar but there is a longitudinal bulging of the abdominal wall in the midline when the patient lifts his head off the bed or coughs, consider *divarication of the recti.*

Finish your examination here

Completion

Tell the examiner you would want to complete the rest of the abdominal examination.

QUESTIONS

(a) What is an epigastric hernia?

A protrusion of extraperitoneal fat (and occasionally peritoneal contents) through a small defect in the linea alba, usually halfway between the xiphoid process and umbilicus.

(b) What symptoms might the patient have complained of at presentation?

The symptoms are commonly confused with other upper gastrointestinal pathologies and include:

- Epigastric pain, which may increase after meals
- May be acutely painful after physical exercise
- Nausea and early satiety
- Reflux and non-ulcer dyspepsia

ADVANCED QUESTIONS

(a) How would you treat this patient?

Non-surgical – the same principles as when managing an incisional hernia (*see* Case 47) would apply. The patient may present with non-specific upper gastrointestinal symptoms; it is particularly important that other causes are considered and ruled out; possible investigations would include:

- Liver function tests and a biliary tree ultrasound scan
- *Helicobacter pylori* serology and upper gastrointestinal endoscopy

Surgical:

- The principles of surgery are that the sac is excised completely or inverted, and the defect in the linea alba repaired
- The fat contained within the hernia can be excised or reduced
- The site of the defect should be marked with the patient lying supine preoperatively, as it may not be possible to find when the patient is anaesthetized

FURTHER READING

Coats R D, Helikson M A, Burd R S (2001) Presentation and management of epigastric hernias in children. *J Pediatr Surg* **35**(12): 1754–6.

www.gensurg.co.uk/epu-epigastric.htm – photographs and diagrams showing epigastric herniae.
www.surgerydoor.co.uk – patient-centred information on how to prepare for over a hundred common operations.

---

* FEMORAL HERNIA   **CASE 74**

INSTRUCTION

'Examine this lady's right groin.'

APPROACH

Expose the patient as for the inguinal hernia examination (Case 42), remembering to examine them lying down if they are presented on a couch, and standing up if they are sitting in a chair (see TOP TIP, Case 42)

VITAL POINTS

These cases appear in the clinical examination very rarely because they are operated on very quickly after presentation, but it is important to know the essential differences from an inguinal hernia and the differential diagnosis of a lump in the groin.

Inspect

- There may be a marble-shaped lump in the groin
- There may be a scar from previous surgery

Palpate

- Identify the anterior superior iliac spine and the pubic tubercle, demonstrating the inguinal ligament between the two (*see* Case 42)
- Femoral herniae are found below the inguinal ligament – compared with inguinal herniae which lie above (Fig. 26)
- Palpate the femoral pulse – the lump lies medial to the pulse
- Ask the patient to cough – femoral herniae usually do not have a cough impulse
- Ask the patient if they can push the lump back – femoral herniae are usually irreducible

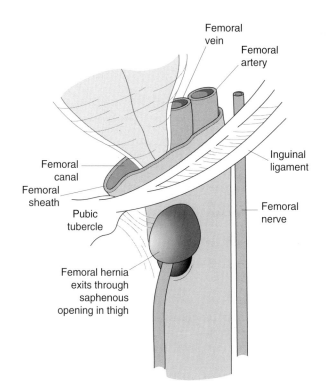

Fig. 26 Femoral hernia.

- Ask if there is any pain and palpate the lump for the characteristic features of a femoral hernia:
  – shape – usually round
  – surface – smooth
  – edge – well defined
  – consistency – firm
  – temperature – same as surrounding skin
  – tenderness – may or may not be tender
  – transilluminability – not transilluminable
  – pulsatility – not pulsatile
  – compressibility – not compressible
  – fluctuance – not fluctuant

Finish your examination here

Completion

Tell the examiner you would examine the contralateral groin for herniae.

QUESTIONS

(a) How can you tell this lump is a femoral hernia (rather than an inguinal hernia)?

See Table 23.

Table 23

Inguinal hernia	Femoral hernia
Above the inguinal ligament	Below the inguinal ligament
Usually reducible	Usually not reducible
M:F 6:1	M:F 1:2 (but note inguinal herniae are still commoner in women than femoral herniae)
Risk of strangulation low	Risk of strangulation high
Cough impulse present	Cough impulse usually absent

(b) What is the differential diagnosis for a femoral hernia?

Skin and soft tissue masses:

- Sebaceous cyst
- Lipoma
- Sarcoma

Vascular masses:

- Saphena varix
- Femoral aneurysm
- Inguinal lymphadenopathy

Other herniae:

- Inguinal hernia
- Obturator hernia (rarely actually palpable)

Others:

- Psoas bursa
- Ectopic testis

ADVANCED QUESTIONS

(a) What are the surgical options for management of a femoral hernia?

The surgical principles are:

- Reduction of the contents of the sac
- Excision of the sac

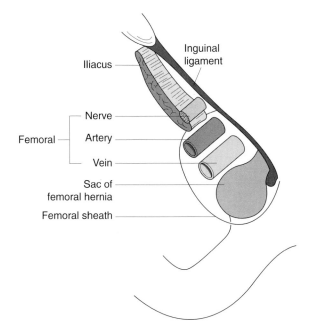

Fig. 27   'NAVY' mnemonic for arrangement of femoral structures (Nerve, Artery, Vein, Y-fronts).

- Repair of the defect – taking care not to narrow the femoral vein while tightening up the femoral canal (Fig. 27)

Possible surgical techniques are:

- Crural or low approach (easiest and most commonly used):
  – an incision is made directly over the hernia, below the medial half of the inguinal ligament
  – the sac is ligated and the femoral canal closed with non-absorbable sutures or a plug
  – best option for elective procedures but risk of narrowing the femoral vein when closing the femoral canal
- Abdominal or preperitoneal repair (McEvedy):
  – Pfannenstiel or lower midline incision is used to repair a bilateral hernia
  – the femoral canal can be closed without breeching the peritoneum
  – best technique for strangulated herniae as it can easily be converted to a more extensive operation seeking any ischaemic bowel without making a second incision
- Inguinal or high repair:
  – the posterior wall of the inguinal canal is opened to access the femoral canal from above
  – best approach if the nature of the hernia is uncertain as inguinal hernias can also be repaired
  – recurrent inguinal hernias are, however, common

FURTHER READING

Cheek C M, Black N A, Devlin H B, Kingsnorth A N, Taylor R S, Watkin D F
(1998) Groin hernia surgery: a systematic review. *Ann R Coll Surg Engl* **80**
(Suppl 1): S1–80 (meta-analysis of results from hernia surgery in the UK).
Chammary V L (1993) Femoral hernia: intestinal obstruction is an unrecognised
source of morbidity and mortality. *Br J Surg* **80**(2): 230–2.

www.vesalius.com/graphics/archive/archtn_her_8.asp – diagrams of the anatomy
of the femoral canal and steps required during operative repair.
www.nlm.nih.gov/medlineplus/ency/article/001136.htm#treatment – patient-
focused discussion of the causes and treatments of femoral hernia.
(These American sites both contain discussions on many other surgical topics too)

MUSCULOSKELETAL AND NEUROLOGY

| CASE 75 | ORTHOPAEDIC HISTORY TAKING – GENERAL APPROACH | *** |

INSTRUCTION

'Ask this patient some questions about her painful hip.'

APPROACH

Occasionally within a short case, and especially in OSCEs, the candidate may be asked to take a history from a patient. In orthopaedics the key elements are:

- Pain
- Loss of function
- Stiffness
- Deformity
- Swelling

VITAL POINTS

Introduction

- Ask the patient's age
- Ask their occupation
- Ask which joints are symptomatic

Pain

- Site – remembering that superficial pain tends to be recognized at the site but pain may be referred, so pain from the hip radiates to the groin, anterior thigh, knee or shin
- Intensity – such as a pain severity score, where the patient allocates a mark out of 10 for the pain
- Frequency – early morning pain is a hallmark of inflammation; pain that is relieved at night is often mechanical in nature; *night pain* is a very important symptom as it indicates the severity of pain and may also raise suspicion of an underlying malignant process
- Analgesic requirement

Loss of function

- Impact on patient's life, e.g. work, sleep

Lower limb:

- Going to the shops
- Use of walking aids, e.g. walking stick(s), Zimmer frame, crutches
- Walking distance (ask them how long or far they can walk before stopping)
- Use of stairs

Upper limb:

- Hand dominance
- Feeding, washing, dressing, brushing hair, writing

Specific to the lumbar spine:

- History of injury
- Radiation of pain – note distribution, particularly looking for dermatomal distribution
- Associated neurological symptoms (e.g. numbness and paraesthesia) and their distribution – the two most commonly involved nerve roots in lumbar disc prolapse are shown in Table 24.

Table 24

Prolapsed disc	Involved nerve root	Distribution of sensory symptoms	Distribution of motor signs	Involved reflexes
L4/L5	L5	Lateral aspect of the leg and dorsum of the foot	Weakness of big toe extension and ankle dorsiflexion	None
L5/S1	S1	Lateral aspect of the foot and heel	Weakness of ankle plantarflexion and foot eversion	Ankle jerk

- Sphincter disturbance – bladder and bowel symptoms secondary to cauda equina compression (unlikely to be present in patients used for examination purposes)

Specific to the hip:

- Assess the stiffness and pain arising from the hip joint
- Ask specifically about ability to:
  – care for their feet/pedicure
  – get in and out of the bath

Specific to the knee:

- Locking of the knee is an intermittent inability to fully extend the knee and suggests a mechanical block – 'Does your knee ever get stuck when you are trying to straighten it?'
- Giving way – a sign of either a patellofemoral problem, loose body, meniscal flap tear or ligamentous laxity – 'Does your knee ever give way when you walk?'

Specific to the feet:

- Ask the patient about back pain (pain at the sole of the foot may be due to a L5/S1 disc prolapse)
- Pins and needles may be due to a lumbar spine pathology, nerve entrapment (such as tarsal tunnel syndrome which is caused by a posterior tibial nerve palsy) or peripheral neuropathy

- Pain present when the patient is barefoot is suggestive of metatarsalgia
- Ask about the patient's shoes – do they have to have special footwear designed?

Past medical history:

- This essentially refers to fitness for surgery/contraindications to anaesthesia in the surgical exam, and the presence of other underlying diseases

CASE 76 — OSTEOARTHRITIS OF THE HIP ★★★

INSTRUCTION

'Examine this lady's right hip.'

APPROACH

- Expose the patient's legs but keep her underwear on
- This examination should be divided clearly into:
  - examining with the patient standing
  - watching the patient walk
  - examining with the patient lying down

VITAL POINTS

Examining with the patient standing (from the front, side and back)

- Comment on the presence of any walking aids
- Look at the hip for scars or sinuses – look particularly for lateral and posterior scars, which are the two most common surgical approaches to the hip
- Look for muscle wasting (particularly the gluteal muscles)
- Look from the side at the patient's posture – increased lumbar lordosis may indicate a fixed flexion deformity at the hip
- Look from the back at the spine – scoliosis may indicate a fixed adduction deformity
- Perform the Trendelenburg test with the patient standing still

Trendelenburg test (Fig. 28)

Ask the patient to stand on her good leg and flex the other leg at the knee as you face her and hold her hands. This manoeuvre is then repeated on the bad leg. The test is positive if the pelvis on the unsupported side (i.e. the side where the leg is flexed) sags down. A positive Trendelenburg test typically occurs in patients with hip abductor weakness – this can be due to chronic hip pain, multiple surgeries, neuromuscular diseases such as polio or underlying structural abnormalities such as developmental hip dysplasia.

A positive Trendelenburg lurch may be also seen in the patient – she throws the upper part of her body over the affected hip in order to compensate for her loss of balance due to the pelvic dip on the contralateral side.

Watching the patient walk

- Begin by asking the patient to stand in front of you
- Watch the patient walk (*see* Case 93) – asking them to walk away from you and then back towards you looking specifically:
  - a Trendelenburg gait, due to abductor weakness (Fig. 28) – characterized by the presence of a sideways lurch of the trunk to bring the patient's body weight over the affected limb
  - an antalgic gait (due to pain) – decreased stance phase and increased swing phase

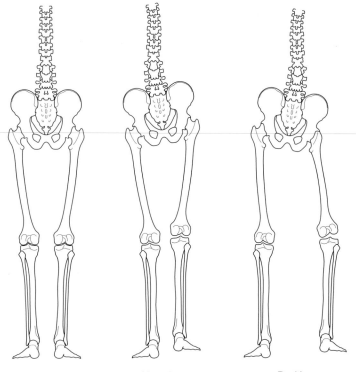

Negative
Trendelenburg test
(normal)

Positive
Trendelenburg test
(abnormal)

Fig. 28 Trendelenburg test.

Examining with the patient lying down

- Ask the patient to lie on the couch
- Measure the real and apparent leg lengths using a tape measure
- This is a difficult concept but one which is frequently asked in the examination
- In both cases, the 'good' leg should be measured first, then the abnormal leg, comparing one side with the other
- The *apparent leg length* is measured from the xiphisternum (a fixed midline bony point) to the medial malleolus while the patient is lying supine with the legs in parallel. With a fixed adduction deformity of the hip, the apparent leg length will be shorter on the affected side, while with a fixed abduction deformity, the apparent leg length will be greater (remembering that you are measuring from the leg to a fixed *midline* point)
- Now ensure that the patient is 'square' on the couch, in other words that they are lying with their pelvis at 90° to the body's long axis. If you are unable to square the pelvis, 'correct' the deformity by placing the normal leg in the same position as the abnormal leg. The *real leg length* is measured from the anterior superior iliac spine to the medial malleolus of the ipsilateral ankle. If different between the two legs, it is due to a 'real' difference in the length of the bones. Real leg length discrepancies can be
  – above the greater trochanter (i.e. in the hip joint) or below it
  – above or below the knee

Palpate

- With the patient still lying down, feel over the greater trochanter for any tenderness (trochanteric bursitis)
- Remember that the joint itself is deep and that the femoral head can only be palpated with deep pressure over the midpoint of the inguinal ligament (*see* Case 42) – this may be uncomfortable for the patient and usually does not add further information

Thomas' test for fixed flexion deformity

- This measures a loss of extension at the hip (a fixed flexion deformity)
- Begin by placing one hand in the small of the patient's back (feeling for lumbar lordosis) and assisting them to flex both their hips and knees as far as possible, feeling for flattening of the lumbar lordosis (Fig. 29)
- Maintain flexion in one hip (ask the patient to hold onto the knee) while asking the patient to extend the other hip as far as possible – by maintaining the flexion of the other hip, the lumbar lordosis is obliterated
- In the presence of any fixed flexion deformity, there will be a point at which further extension ceases and the residual flexion (fixed flexion) is measured from the horizontal
- Repeat with the other leg
- These movements can also be combined with measuring range of movement of the hips in a 'cycling' manoeuvre

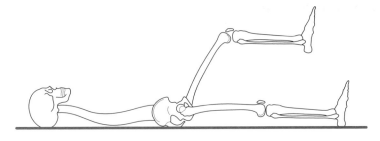

Normal

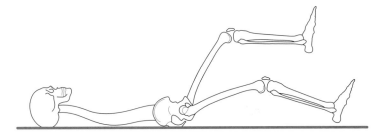

Positive Thomas test:
fixed flexion deformity in right hip

Fig. 29 Thomas' test.

Movements of the hip

Carefully watch the patient's face at all times during this examination and be sure to ask the patient to tell you if there is any discomfort before attempting any passive joint movements.

- Assess each muscle group in turn, remembering that the movements of the hip are flexion/extension, abduction/adduction and internal/external rotation (see Table 25)
- Begin by asking the patient to flex the hip up to the anterior abdominal wall with the knee flexed, measuring the angle of active flexion
- Stress the flexed hip more to see whether there is any further passive flexion
- At this point, the Thomas' test can be performed too (see above)
- Bring the hip back to 90° of flexion, at right angles to the couch. Keeping the knees flexed, measure internal and external rotation
- Finally ask the patient to straighten the leg again and, with the hip fully extended, measure abduction and adduction. Detect any tilting of the pelvis by placing one hand on one of the anterior superior iliac spines (it does not matter which one)
- You can also measure internal and external rotation with the knee in extension by comparing movements of the patella (Table 25)

Table 25 Movements of the hip

Hip movement	Muscle group	Expected movement
Flexion	Iliopsoas, rectus femoris, tensor fascia lata, quads	140°
Extension	Gluteus maximus and hamstrings	10°
Abduction	Gluteus medius and minimus	45°
Adduction	Adductors (longus, brevis, magnus)	30°
Internal rotation	Gluteus medius, minimus, iliopsoas	40°
External rotation	Gluteus maximus	40°

Finish your examination here

Completion

Tell the examiner you would:

- Examine the back and knee (the joints above and below the hip, as pain in one joint may be referred to the next)
- Examine the neurology of the limb
- Examine the vascular supply of the limb
- Offer to help the patient to dress

QUESTIONS

(a) How should this patient be investigated?

There is no specific laboratory test for osteoarthritis – usually the diagnosis is made with a combination of clinical features and X-ray appearances. However, tests are performed to exclude other systemic diseases that may cause hip pain, particularly rheumatological and collagen-vascular disorders:

Blood tests include:
- Haematological – full blood count, erythrocyte sedimentation rate
- Biochemical – baseline renal and liver function, particularly if long-term nonsteroidal anti-inflammatory medication is being considered
- Immunological – rheumatoid factor, antinuclear antibody

Radiological tests used are plain anteroposterior and lateral X-rays of the hip and pelvis.

(b) What are the X-ray features of osteoarthritis of the hip?

Use the mnemonic **LOSS** to remember these features:

L Loss of the joint space
O Osteophyte formation
S Subchondral sclerosis
S Subchondral cysts

(c) What are the treatment options?

This is a 'classic' examination question which should be answered in a clearly structured way.

Non-surgical options would include:

- Lifestyle modifications – diet and exercise are important, including weight loss if appropriate, and patients may need referral to appropriate services
- Physiotherapy – some patients will respond to personalized exercise regimens which will improve their symptoms and may delay the need for a total hip replacement
- Occupational therapy – fitting of suitable devices to aid mobility (such as walking sticks, frames, etc) and more importantly practical advice on how to use them
- Medical therapy – using the pain ladder (*see* Case 118) beginning with paracetamol and non-steroidal anti-inflammatories

Surgical options include:

- Osteotomy
- Arthroplasty (i.e. hip replacement)
- Arthrodesis

The US National Institute of Health concluded in 1994 that the indications for total hip replacement are:

- Instability
- Severe pain or disability that is not substantially relieved by an extended course of non-surgical management
- Rest pain or pain with movement
- Loss of mobility

ADVANCED QUESTIONS

(a) What are the complications of total hip replacement?

Complications can be divided into intraoperative, immediate (within 24 hours), early (within 30 days) and late (later than 30 days). Specific complications include:

Intraoperative:

- Perforation or fracture of the acetabulum or femur

Immediate:

- Dislocation (due to incorrect placement of the prosthetic components)

Early:

- Deep vein thrombosis (DVT) and pulmonary embolus (PE)
- Sciatic nerve palsy (more common in the posterior surgical approach to the hip joint)
- Infection
- Fat embolism syndrome

Late:

- Infection
- Loosening (septic or aseptic)
- Heterotopic ossification
- Leg-length discrepancy
- Periprosthetic fractures
- Thigh pain

(b) How do you prevent postoperative deep vein thrombosis following a total hip replacement?

DVT is the commonest complication following total hip replacement, with a peak incidence at 5–10 days postoperatively

Prevention is impossible but measures that can be taken are classified according to

- PREOPERATIVE: Thromboembolic deterrent (TED) stockings fitted preoperatively
- PERIOPERATIVE: TED stockings, minimising the length of surgery, using compression boots and foot pumps
- POSTOPERATIVE: low dose or low molecular weight heparin can reduce incidence of DVT, early mobilisation of patients with the help of physiotherapists

> *Friedrich Trendelenburg (1844–1924).* Professor of Surgery, Bonn and Leipzig, Germany.
> *H.O. Thomas (1834–1891).* General Practitioner in Liverpool who founded orthopaedic services in the city and also designed a range of splints as he believed in the power of complete rest to heal fractures – many of these were used in the First World War

FURTHER READING

Hoaglund F T, Steinbach L S (2001) Primary osteoarthritis of the hip: etiology and epidemiology. *J Am Acad Orthop Surg* **9**(5): 320–7.

Turpie A G C, Levine M, Hirsch J (1986) A randomized controlled trial of a low-molecular weight heparin (enoxaparin) to prevent deep vein thrombosis in patients undergoing elective hip surgery. *N Engl J Med* **315**: 925–9.

http://www.medmedia.com/oa4/14.htm – online textbook with in-depth information about osteoarthritis

*** **OSTEOARTHRITIS OF THE KNEE**   CASE 77

INSTRUCTION

'Examine this gentleman's right knee.'

APPROACH

Adequately expose both lower limbs, keeping the gentleman's underwear on.

VITAL POINTS

Inspect with the patient standing (front and back)

- Comment on the presence of any walking aids
- Shape:
  - alignment – is the knee in varus or valgus (you can measure intermalleolar distance if the examiner asks you to quantify this) or is there fixed flexion or hyperextension present? Look particularly for varus and fixed flexion deformities in patients with osteoarthritis
  - obvious quadriceps wasting?
- Scars – look particularly for:
  - arthroscopic portal scars (*see* Case 90)
  - meniscectomy scars (*see* Case 90)
  - total or unicondylar knee replacement scars – midline longitudinal incision
- Swellings – especially popliteal fossa ?Baker's cyst (*see* Case 95)

Gait (*see* Case 93)

- Antalgic – if the knee is painful – seen in osteoarthritis
- Stiff knee gait – pelvis rises to allow the leg clearance during the swing phase – seen in severe osteoarthritis
- Instability (thrust) gait – may be mechanical or neuropathic

Ask the patient to lie down on the couch

Measure

- Quadriceps wasting – measure thigh circumference at a set distance (e.g. 15 cm) above the superior pole of the patella and compare with the opposite side

Feel

- Temperature – using the dorsum of the hand from the proximal thigh to the distal leg
- Tenderness – start with the knee in extension and feel around the margins of the patella:

- grind test – move patella up and down while pressing it gently against the femur – painful grating is indicative of patellofemoral compartment pathology, e.g. patellofemoral osteoarthritis (PFOA)
- Clarke's test – press the patella backwards and distally onto the patellofemoral groove, and ask the patient to gently contract his quadriceps muscle – pain at this point is indicative of patellofemoral compartment pathology, e.g. PFOA

- Next flex the knee to 90° and ensure the foot is flat on the couch
  - feel the lateral and medial joint lines of the knee (there may be tenderness at the joint line of involved compartments in osteoarthritis)
  - feel the posterior aspect of the knee for any popliteal fossa swellings (*see* Case 95)

- Effusion:
  - patellar hollow test (for very small quantities of fluid) – as the normal knee is flexed, a hollow appears lateral to the patellar tendon and disappears with further flexion – with intraarticular fluid, the hollow fills and disappears at lesser angles of flexion – you may even notice that the hollows have disappeared altogether compared with the normal knee
  - bulge test (for small quantities of fluid) – empty the medial compartment by pressing on that side of the joint, then sharply swipe across the lateral aspect of the knee and observe for a ripple or bulge to appear on the medial aspect of the knee
  - patellar tap (for moderate amounts of fluid) – compress the suprapatellar pouch with your left hand, and use the index finger of your right hand to push the patella sharply backwards – the patella can be felt to hit the femoral condyles and to bounce off
  - cross-fluctuation (for large quantities of fluid) – use your left hand to compress and empty the suprapatellar pouch, and with your right hand, empty the medial side of the knee by sweeping the back of the hand up the medial side, then sweep down the lateral side and observe the fluid impulse transmitted across the joint

Move

- Extension – ask the patent to press his thigh into the couch and note any presence of hyperextension (if no hyperextension, the range of movement is 0° extension)
- Flexion – normally the knee flexes until the calf meets the hamstring – this is around 140° – during this movement, place your hand over the patella and note any clicks or crepitus
- You may elicit a fixed flexion deformity and decreased flexion in patients with osteoarthritis – the movements may also be painful, so it is important to be very gentle

Special tests

This is part of the routine knee examination and should be carried out in the exam unless the examiner stops you. In patients with osteoarthritis, the most common finding with these tests is a degenerate meniscal tear, which may give you a positive McMurray's test.

- Cruciate ligaments (ensure that the quadriceps and hamstrings are relaxed):
  - posterior sag – flex both knees to 90°, keeping the feet flat on the couch, and look across at the anterior profile of both knees – if there is a 'drop back' or sag of the upper end of the tibia, or the upper end can be gently pushed back, this indicates a tear of the posterior cruciate ligament (PCL) (the 'sag sign')
  - anterior drawer – flex the knee to 90° and sit on the foot to stabilize it (ensuring that the foot is not tender), then use both hands to pull the upper end of the tibia forwards (= anterior drawer). A positive test indicates an anterior cruciate ligament (ACL) injury. The test can be graded according to the distance forward that the tibia moves (1+ = 0 – 5 mm, 2+ = 6 – 10 mm, 3+ = 11 – 15 mm and 4+ = > 15 mm) and according to the feel of the endpoint of the movement (firm = ACL intact, marginal or soft). Note that positive posterior sag can give you a false-positive anterior drawer test
  - posterior drawer – performed in a similar manner to the anterior drawer test except that the upper end of the tibia is pushed backwards. A positive test is indicative of a PCL injury. It is graded in a similar manner to the anterior drawer test
  - Lachman's test (most sensitive for ACL injury) – flex the knee to 20° and holding distal thigh firmly with your left hand, lift the proximal tibia forward with your right hand with your thumb on the anteromedial joint line. If you find this difficult, either because you have small hands or the patient has big thighs, an alternative method is to flex the patient's knee over your thigh, press down on the distal thigh of the patient and lift the proximal tibia forward. The test can be graded according to the distance forward that the tibia moves and according to the feel of the endpoint of the movement, as in the anterior drawer test
- Collateral ligaments:
  - tuck the patient's foot under your arm and flex the knee to 20–30°, then apply valgus and varus stresses to the knee alternately while feeling the joint line for opening. The test can be alternatively performed by using the left hand to hold the knee and the right hand to hold the ankle, although this does require more strength. Opening of the medial joint line on valgus stress testing signifies a medial collateral ligament injury, while opening of the lateral joint line on varus stress testing signifies a lateral collateral ligament injury
  - repeat the varus and valgus stress test with the knee in full extension. Instability in extension signifies a combined collateral and cruciate ligament injury
- Menisci:
  - McMurray's test – this test, if done accurately, can help to differentiate between medial and lateral meniscal tears, but often does not add much information to your clinical examination. Flex the knee maximally, and grasp the knee with one hand and the foot with the other. To test the medial meniscus, palpate the posteromedial joint line and externally rotate the leg and for the lateral meniscus, palpate the posterolateral joint line and internally rotate the leg. Now slowly extend the knee and feel for a palpable

click, which is indicative of a meniscal tear. Pain during the test is also suggestive of a meniscal tear. It is also said that a click that is palpable from moving from full flexion to 90° flexion is suggestive of a posterior tear of the meniscus, while a click that is palpable moving from 90° flexion to full extension is suggestive of a middle or anterior tear of the meniscus. The test can also be repeated with valgus (testing medial meniscus) and varus (testing lateral meniscus) stresses applied

Finish your examination here

Completion

Say that you would like to:

- Examine the hip and ankle (the joints above and below the knee joint)
- Assess the neurovascular status of the limb
- Ask the patient some questions to ascertain how much the problem affects his life, particularly activities of daily living, the presence of night pain and his mobility

QUESTIONS

(a) What are the X-ray changes of osteoarthritis of the knee?

Remember the mnemonic **LOSS** for radiological features of osteoarthritis:

L Loss of the joint space
O Osteophyte formation
S Subchondral sclerosis
S Subchondral cysts

More specifically, ensure that the X-rays have been taken with the patient standing and bearing weight, so that even small degrees of articular cartilage thinning can be seen. The tibiofemoral joint space is diminished (usually medial compartment) and the lateral X-ray may show patellofemoral osteoarthritis. There may also be soft-tissue calcification in the suprapatellar region or in the joint – this is known as chondrocalcinosis.

(b) How do you treat osteoarthritis of the knee?

Non-surgical:

- Lifestyle modifications – diet and exercise are important, including weight-loss if appropriate, and patients may need referral to appropriate services
- Physiotherapy – many patients will respond to personalized exercise regimens that will improve their symptoms and may delay for many years the need for a knee replacement. Strengthening the quadriceps muscles is very important
- Occupational therapy – fitting of suitable devices to aid mobility (such as walking sticks, frames, etc) and more importantly practical advice on how to use them. Even a simple elastic support may help, probably by improving proprioception in an unstable knee

- Medical therapy – using the pain ladder (*see* Case 118) beginning with paracetamol and non-steroidal anti-inflammatories
- Intra-articular steroid injections – may provide temporary relief, but repeated injections may lead to progressive cartilage and bone destruction
- Viscosupplementation – intra-articular injections of hyaluronic acid may provide benefit, but they are not in widespread use due to their expense and the presence of side-effects

Surgical options include:

- Arthroscopic debridement and washout – may give temporary relief and is of use in younger patients as a temporizing procedure before subsequent arthroplasty; degenerate meniscal tears and osteophytes can be trimmed
- Patellectomy – indicated in rare cases where osteoarthritis is confined only to the patellofemoral joint; may result in decreased extensor mechanism power, and if total knee replacement is needed later results in less predictable pain relief
- Realignment osteotomy – useful particularly in younger patients (under 50 years) with medial compartment osteoarthritis, in whom a high tibial valgus osteotomy redistributes weight to the lateral side of the joint
- Unicompartmental or total knee arthroplasty (i.e. knee replacement) – indicated in older patients with progressive joint destruction. If the disease is confined to one compartment, a unicompartmental knee replacement can be performed as an alternative to osteotomy.
- Arthrodesis – indicated if there is a strong contraindication to arthroplasty (e.g. previous sepsis) or as a salvage procedure for a failed arthroplasty

QUESTION

What are the complications of a total knee replacement?

Intraoperative:

- Fracture of the tibia or femur

Immediate:

- Vascular injuries – superficial femoral, popliteal and genicular vessels

Early:

- Deep vein thrombosis (DVT) and pulmonary embolus (PE)
- Peroneal nerve palsy (1%)
- Infection
- Fat embolism syndrome

Late:

- Infection
- Loosening (septic or aseptic)
- Patellar instability/fractures/disruption of extensor mechanism
- Periprosthetic fractures

ADVANCED QUESTIONS

(a) Rheumatoid arthritis is another disease that can affect the knee. What do you know of the clinical features of rheumatoid arthritis of the knee?

Stage 1 – proliferative:

- Palpable effusions and thickened synovium but stable joint
- Posterior capsule at risk of rupture
- Acute rupture of Baker's cysts (*see* Case 95)

Stage 2 – destructive:

- Increasing instability of the knee joint
- Marked muscle wasting
- Some loss of flexion and extension

Stage 3 – reparative:

- Severe pain and instability – there may be marked stiffness or severe instability
- Commonest deformities are fixed flexion and valgus
- Instability manifests as increased anteroposterior glide and lateral wobble

(b) What are the surgical options for rheumatoid arthritis of the knee?

- Synovectomy and debridement – for failed medical treatment. This procedure can be performed arthroscopically and involves removing the articular pannus and cartilage
- Supracondylar osteotomy – useful if the knee is stable and pain-free but troubled by valgus and flexion deformity
- Total knee arthroplasty – for advanced joint destruction

FURTHER READING

Cole B J, Harner C D (1999) Degenerative arthritis of the knee in active patients: evaluation and management. *J Am Acad Orthop Surg* **7**(6): 389–402

Stuart M J (1999) Arthroscopic management for degenerative arthritis of the knee. *Instr Course Lect* **48**: 135–41

http://www.aafp.org/afp/20000315/1795.html – a very useful online paper published by the American Family Physician with approaches to managing hip and knee osteoarthritis

*** DUPUYTREN'S CONTRACTURE CASE 78

INSTRUCTION

'Examine this patient's hands.'

APPROACH

Expose to elbows and ask the patient to place his hands palm upwards on a pillow (if available).

VITAL POINTS

Look

- Describe any tethering or pitting of the skin on the palmar aspect of the hand, and also note the appearance of any visible cords
- Look for scars from previous surgery
- Describe any flexion deformities at the metacarpophalangeal and proximal interphalangeal joints (MCPJ and PIPJ) of the involved fingers
- Look for involvement of the thumb and the first web space (a sign of more aggressive disease)
- Ask the patient to turn his hands over to look for Garrod's pads (thickening of the subcutaneous tissues) over the PIPJ

Feel

- Palpate the swelling, particularly noting its fixation to skin
- Does the other palm have similar thickening?

Move

- Assess the range of motion in the involved fingers
- Note the presence of fixed deformities by passively moving the involved joints

> TOP TIP
>
> Asking the patient to lay the involved hand flat against a hard surface, e.g. a table may facilitate assessment of the deformities and allow you to judge the extent to which they are fixed (*table-top test*).

Finish your examination here

Completion

Say that you would like to:

- Enquire about causes and associations (see below)
- Assess the patient's function, e.g. writing and dressing
- Look for other features of diffuse fibromatosis

QUESTIONS

(a) What is your differential diagnosis?

The differential diagnosis includes:

- Skin contracture – look for scar from previous wound
- Tendon contracture – thickened area, which *moves* on passive flexion of involved finger
- Congenital contracture of the little finger – affects PIPJ
- Ulnar nerve palsy – ring and little fingers are hyperextended at MCPJ and flexed at PIPJ

(b) What conditions are associated with Dupuytren's contracture?

We have found the following mnemonic helpful to remember the associations – **DEAFEST PAIL**:

Diabetes mellitus
Epilepsy
Age (positive correlation)
Family history (autosomal dominant)/**F**ibromatoses*
Epileptic medication (e.g. phenobarbitone)
Smoking
Trauma and heavy manual labour
Peyronie's disease (fibrosis of the corpus cavernosum – seen in 3% of patients with Dupuytren's)
AIDS
Idiopathic (most common)
Liver disease (secondary to alcohol)

*A group of disorders characterized by diffuse fibrosis, which include such diverse conditions as desmoid tumours, Reidel's thyroiditis, retroperitoneal fibrosis and Ledderhose disease (fibrosis of the *plantar* aponeurosis – seen in 5% of patients with Dupuytren's)

(c) What are the surgical options available?

Operative management is considered when MCPJ or PIPJ contracture exceeds 30°:

- Fasciotomy – for prominent bands
- Partial fasciectomy (with Z-plasty to lengthen wound) – in conjunction with postoperative physiotherapy (early active-flexion range-of-motion exercises for grip strength) and night-time splintage in extension
- Dermofasciectomy (with full-thickness skin grafting) – associated with the lowest risk of recurrence
- Arthrodesis/amputation – for late presentations and repeated recurrences

ADVANCED QUESTIONS

(a) What is the underlying pathophysiology of the condition?

Local microvessel ischaemia is thought to result in increased activity of xanthine oxidase, resulting in superoxide free radical production that in turn stimulates myofibroblast proliferation and type III collagen formation. Specific platelet-derived and fibroblast growth factors also play a role in the aetiology. Allopurinol, which inhibits xanthine oxidase, may help to reduce symptoms.

The process of chronic inflammation is thought to be essential to the subsequent fibrosis (see Further reading).

Baron Guillaume Dupuytren (1777–1835) – Surgeon in Chief, Hotel-Dieu, Paris. He described the condition as 'permanent retraction of the fingers' and was also Surgeon to Louis XVIII and Charles X during the restoration of the Bourbon monarchy. He was a cold, rude, ambitious and arrogant man, earning him the epithet 'the Napoleon of Surgery'. He died following a stroke and was described as 'first among surgeons; last among men'.

Sir A. E. Garrod (1857–1936) – English Physician, St. Bartholomew's Hospital, London, later succeeding William Osler as Regius Professor at Oxford

G. Ledderhose (1855–1925) – German Surgeon

Francois Gigot de la Peyronie (1678–1747) – French Surgeon

FURTHER READING

Saar J D, Grothaus P C (2000) Dupuytren's disease: an overview. *Plast Reconstr Surg* **106**(1): 125–34

Meek R M D, McLellan, Crossan J F (1999) Dupuytren's disease. *J Bone Joint Surg Br* 81B: 732–8

Benson L S, Williams C S, Kahle M (1998) Dupuytren's contracture. *J Am Acad Orthop Surg* **6**(1): 24–35

www.gh.vic.gov.au/periop/gensurg/dupuytre.htm – patient-centred information

CASE 79	CARPAL TUNNEL SYNDROME * * *

INSTRUCTION

'This lady is complaining of a tingling sensation in the thumb and index fingers of the right hand. Examine her hands and tell me what you think the diagnosis is.'

APPROACH

Expose to elbows and ask the patient to place her hands palm upwards on a pillow (if available).

VITAL POINTS

The clues are in the instruction. The examiner is expecting you to perform a *directed* neurological assessment of the hands. He is leading you towards to the diagnosis with his question, but is interested in seeing how you approach the task.

Look

- Wasting of the thenar muscles (in advanced cases)
- Scar from previous surgery over the transverse carpal ligament

Sensory assessment

Test light touch over the palmar aspects of the thumb, index and middle fingers of the involved hand – deficiency implies median nerve involvement. Compare this with the other fingers, proceeding to other sensory modalities such as pain only if the examiner wishes you to.

TOP TIP 1

The autonomous sensory areas of the hand (i.e. only one nerve always supplies this area) are as follows:

- Median nerve – distal phalanges of index and middle fingers
- Ulnar nerve – middle and distal phalanges of little finger
- Radial nerve – over first dorsal interosseus muscle between first and second metacarpals (but usually there is no autonomous zone)

Testing these three areas confirms restriction of pathology to one nerve only

---

Motor assessment

Test the power of muscles innervated by the median nerve (**LOAF**) (Fig. 30):

Lateral two **l**umbricals – difficult to test
Opponens pollicis – oppose the patient's thumb and the little finger and ask her to stop you pulling the fingers apart

Abductor pollicis brevis – place dorsum of hand on a flat surface and ask the patient to lift her thumb to the ceiling against resistance

Flexor pollicis brevis – not an autonomous muscle (innervation varies).

Test only for abductor pollicis brevis in the exam (see Top Tip 2)

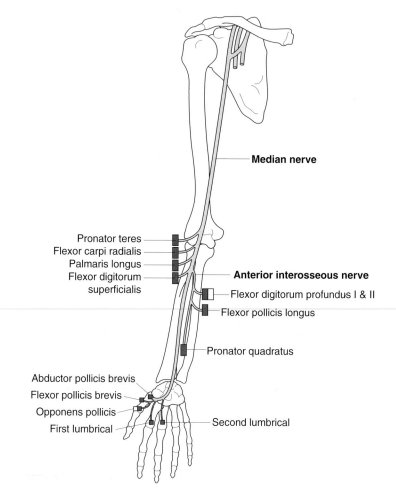

Pronator teres
Flexor carpi radialis
Palmaris longus
Flexor digitorum superficialis

Median nerve

Anterior interosseous nerve

Flexor digitorum profundus I & II
Flexor pollicis longus

Pronator quadratus

Abductor pollicis brevis
Flexor pollicis brevis
Opponens pollicis
First lumbrical

Second lumbrical

Fig. 30 Muscles supplied by the median nerve.

TOP TIP 2

The autonomous motor supply of the hand are:

- Median nerve – abductor pollicis brevis (as above)
- Ulnar nerve – palmar interossei (adduction of the fingers)
- Radial nerve – metacarpophalangeal extensors (extension of the fingers at the knuckles)

Finish your examination here

Completion

Say that you would like to perform the following special tests:

- Tinel's sign – tapping over the median nerve at the wrist reproduces tingling sensation in the distribution of the nerve
- Phalen's test – maximal flexion of the wrist for 1 minute exacerbates symptoms which are promptly relieved when flexion is discontinued
- Flexion compression test (also known as Duran's test) – maximal flexion of wrist and direct digital compression of the median nerve at the wrist reproduces symptoms (if symptoms appear within 20 sec, sensitivity = 82% and specificity = 99%)

Assess the effect of the symptoms on the patient's quality of life, e.g. symptoms are usually worse at night and first thing in the morning – sleep quality may be affected.

Look for underlying causes and associations (see below).

QUESTIONS

(a) What are the causes of carpal tunnel syndrome?

The most common cause is *idiopathic*. The other causes can be classified as follows:

- Anatomical abnormalities:
  - bone – previous wrist fractures, e.g. Colles fracture, acromegaly
  - soft tissues – lipomas, ganglia
- Physiological abnormalities:
  - inflammatory conditions – rheumatoid arthritis, gout
  - alterations of fluid balance – pregnancy, menopause, hypothyroidism, obesity, amyloidosis, renal failure
  - neuropathic conditions – diabetes mellitus, alcoholism

(b) Name one investigation you might perform before offering this lady treatment?

Nerve conduction studies:

- Symptoms of carpal tunnel syndrome can be mimicked by higher (more proximal) lesions of the median nerve. These high lesions are characterized by loss of sensation over the thenar eminence due to involvement of the palmar cutaneous branch, and loss of the relevant forearm flexors (especially flexor pollicis longus)
- Symptoms may also be due to cervical nerve root lesions (e.g. secondary to a cervical disc herniation) or thoracic outlet syndrome
- Nerve conduction studies also assist in determining the severity of the lesion

(c) How would you treat this lady?

- Non-surgical – removal of underlying causes, splinting of the wrist in a neutral position (especially at night-time), and local steroid injections just proximal to the carpal tunnel

- Surgical – carpal tunnel decompression (division of the flexor retinaculum under tourniquet control) can be performed either as an open or endoscopic procedure

(d) What complications would you warn this lady about if you were offering her surgery?

- Scar formation – high-risk area for keloid or hypertrophic scars
- Scar tenderness – can occur in up to 40% of patients
- Wound infection
- Nerve injury – palmar cutaneous branch of the median nerve (which lies superficial to the retinaculum) and the motor branch to the thenar muscles (which usually leaves the radial side of the median nerve towards the distal extent of the standard incision). The risk of nerve injury is decreased if the skin incision is made on the ulnar side of the palmar crease
- Failure to relieve symptoms – if the retinaculum is incompletely divided

ADVANCED QUESTIONS

(a) What are the boundaries of the carpal tunnel?

- Ulnar aspect – pisiform (where flexor carpi ulnaris attaches) and hook of hamate
- Radial aspect – scaphoid and trapezium
- Volar aspect – transverse carpal ligament

(b) Where else is the median nerve likely to be compressed?

The following causes are rare:

- Pronator syndrome – compression of the median nerve by the ligament of Struthers (fibrous band arising from the medial epicondyle of the humerus that passes medially and upwards to attach to a supratrochlear spur on the lower anterior humerus), pronator teres muscle or the proximal arch of the flexor digitorum superficialis
- Anterior interosseous syndrome – entrapment of the anterior interosseous branch of the median nerve, usually at the origin of the deep head of pronator teres. The nerve supplies flexor pollicis longus, pronator quadratus and the radial side of flexor digitorum profundus, leading to loss of precise pinch (inability to make the 'OK sign'), but there are *no* sensory signs

(c) What is the pathophysiology underlying carpal tunnel syndrome (or any compression syndrome)?

The primary change is thought to be vascular in origin. Pressure on the nerve results in blood-flow obstruction in the vasa nervorum, resulting in venous congestion and oedema. With time, fibroblast proliferation occurs in the nerve, leading to inefficiency of cell transport mechanisms and the sodium pump, resulting in impairment of nerve conduction.

> *Jules Tinel (1879–1952)* – French neurologist
> *George S Phalen* – American Orthopaedic Surgeon, worked at the Cleveland Clinic in Ohio

FURTHER READING

Kanaan N, Sawaya R A (2001) Carpal tunnel syndrome: modern diagnostic and management techniques. *Br J Gen Pract* **51**(465): 311–4

Jimenez D F, Gibbs S R, Clapper A T (1998) Endoscopic treatment of carpal tunnel syndrome: a critical review. *J Neurosurg* **88**(5): 817–26

Cantatore F P, Dell'Accio F, Lapadula G (1997) Carpal tunnel syndrome: a review. *Clin Rheumatol* **16**(6): 596–603

Baguneid M S, Sochart D H, Dunlop D, Kenny N W (1997) Carpal tunnel decompression under local anaesthetic and tourniquet control. *Br J Hand Surg* **22**(3): 322–4

http://www.medicalmultimediagroup.com/pated/ctd/cts/cts.html – guide to carpal tunnel syndrome for patients

CASE 80   RHEUMATOID HANDS   ★★★

INSTRUCTION

'Examine this lady's hands.'

APPROACH

Expose the hands and the forearms to the elbows (to examine for rheumatoid nodules later in the case) and place on a white pillow or blanket, palm upwards.

VITAL POINTS

Almost all the clinical signs are elicited on inspection alone.

Look

Wrist:

- Radial deviation of the wrist
- Volar subluxation of the wrist joint
- Piano-key sign – subluxation of the radio-ulnar joint causes the head of the ulna to pop up on the dorsum of the wrist where it can be jogged up and down

Thumb:

- The 'Z-thumb' appearance, with flexion of the interphalangeal joint and hyperextension of the metacarpophalangeal joint (MCPJ)

Palm:

- The presence of palmar erythema

Fingers:

- Ulnar deviation of the fingers, involving the more lateral digits in more advanced cases
- Metacarpophalangeal joint volar subluxation, most commonly over the index and middle fingers
- Swelling of the proximal interphalangeal joints (PIPJ)
- Swan neck deformity (flexion of the DIPJ and hyperextension of the PIPJ) (Fig. 31)
- Boutonniere deformity (hyperextension of the DIPJ and flexion of the PIPJ) (Fig. 31)

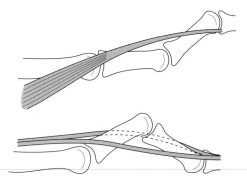

Fig. 31 Swan neck (above) and boutonniere (below) deformities of the rheumatoid hand.

Dorsum:

- Wasting of the interossei, best seen in the first dorsal webspace

Palpate

- Palpate over any swollen joints to detect the warmth and tenderness of acutely inflamed joints
- Finally palpate the elbows (over the subcutaneous border of the ulna) for rheumatoid nodules – present in 25% of patients, especially in active seropositive disease. You may also find rheumatoid nodules at other pressure areas, e.g. the pulps of the fingers and the radial side of the index finger

Sensory and motor assessment

See the section under carpal tunnel syndrome (Case 79) – the median nerve may be involved in rheumatoid arthritis if carpal tunnel syndrome is a complication.

Functional assessment

Ask the patient to perform simple tests such as unbuttoning a shirt and writing with a pen, in order to assess the function of the hands, and determine the need for specific treatments.

Finish your examination here

Completion

Tell the examiner that you would wish to:

- Ask the patient what other joints in the body are affected by rheumatoid arthritis
- Examine the rest of the patient for other features of rheumatoid arthritis (see below)
- Ask the patient how the condition affects her life

QUESTIONS

(a) What are the extra-articular manifestations of rheumatoid arthritis?

Ophthalmic:

- Episcleritis
- Scleritis
- Keratoconjuctivitis sicca

Respiratory:

- Pleural effusions
- Pulmonary fibrosis

Cardiac:

- Pericarditis

Reticuloendothelial:

- Lymphadenopathy
- Splenomegaly
- Felty's syndrome (*see* Case 49)

Neurological:

- Multifocal neuropathies
- Carpal tunnel syndrome

Vascular:

- Vasculitis

(b) What investigations can be used to confirm the diagnosis of rheumatoid arthritis?

Blood tests:

- Haematological
  - anaemia of chronic disease (due to decreased production of red blood cells, increased destruction of red cells or ineffective erythropoiesis)
  - raised erythrocyte sedimentation rate
- Immunological
  - rheumatoid factor is positive in 75%
  - HLA-DR3/DR4 present in approximately one-third of patients
  - anti nuclear antibody (ANA) is raised in 30%

X-rays (see below).

(c) What are the treatment options for rheumatoid arthritis?

Non-surgical (hand therapy/physiotherapy):

- Splinting (static and dynamic)
- Active hand and wrist exercises
- Household aids and personal aids (orthoses)

Injections – local injections of corticosteroid and local anaesthetic for persistent synovitis of a few joints or tendon sheaths.

Pharmacological:

- First-line drug treatment with non-steroidal anti-inflammatory drugs (considering the need for a gastric mucosal protective agent such as the addition of a proton pump inhibitor, or a prostaglandin analogue such as misoprostol) or COX-2 inbibitors which specifically inhibit cyclooxygenase 2, reducing the incidence of gastrointestinal bleeding (which is mediated through COX-1)
- Second-line treatment is with sulphasalazine, hydroxychloroquine, or penicillamine
- Third-line treatment, to prevent disease progression, includes gold or low-dose methotrexate

Surgical:

- Operative options include soft tissue procedures (e.g. synovectomy, carpal tunnel decompression and tendon repairs/transfers) and bone/joint procedures (e.g. arthrodesis and arthroplasty). You would not be expected to know the details for MRCS

ADVANCED QUESTIONS

(a) What are the clinical stages of rheumatoid arthritis of the hand?

- Stage 1 – proliferative – synovitis of the joints (swelling of MCPJ and PIPJ) and of tendon sheaths (flexor and extensor tenosynovitis, the former leading to carpal tunnel syndrome)

- Stage 2 – destructive – joint and tendon erosions, e.g. drop finger and mallet thumb due to extensor tendon ruptures, radial deviation of the wrist and ulnar deviation of the fingers
- Stage 3 – reparative – leading to established deformities such as marked ulnar deviation of the fingers, volar dislocation of the MCPJs, and multiple swan-neck and boutonniere deformities

(b) What are the radiological stages of rheumatoid arthritis?

- Stage 1 – soft tissue swelling and periarticular osteoporosis
- Stage 2 – joint space narrowing and small periarticular erosions (most common at MCPJs and styloid process of the ulna)
- Stage 3 – marked articular destruction, seen most commonly at MCPJs, PIPJs and wrist joints

FURTHER READING

Ollivier J E (2001) Advances in the management of osteoarthritis and rheumatoid arthritis. *JAAPA* **14**(10): 22–5, 29–30, 36–8

Davidson A, Diamond B (2001) Autoimmune diseases. *N Engl J Med* **345**(5): 340–50

http://www.arthritis.ca/types%20of%20arthritis/ra/default.asp?s=1 – patient information on rheumatoid arthritis from The Arthritis Society

CASE 81	OSTEOARTHITIS IN THE HANDS ★★★

INSTRUCTION

'Examine this gentleman's hands.'

APPROACH

Expose the hands and the forearms to the elbows and place on a white pillow or blanket, palm upwards.

VITAL POINTS

Almost all the clinical signs are elicited on inspection alone.

Look

- The distal interphalangeal joints (DIPJ) are swollen (Heberden's nodes) and may be fixed in flexion
- Bouchard's nodes are bony swellings at the proximal interphalangeal joints (PIPJ) in osteoarthritis
- 'Square hand' appearance – see below

Palpate

- Continue to test *active* and *passive* movements of the affected joints to define degree of reduction of movement.

Functional assessment

Ask the patient to perform simple tests such as unbuttoning a shirt, in order to assess the function of the hands.

Finish your examination here

Completion

Tell the examiner that you would wish to examine other joints for arthritis. In comparison with rheumatoid arthritis, the hips, lumbar spine and knees are more commonly affected than the hands.

QUESTIONS

(a) Which joints in the hands are most frequently affected by osteoarthritis?

- DIPJ (Heberden's nodes)
- PIPJ (Bouchard's nodes) – these are strongly associated with polyarticular osteoarthritis, i.e. arthritis at other joints in the body, including carpometacarpal arthritis
- Carpo-metacarpal joint (CMCJ) of the thumb – which sometimes leads to the 'square hand' or 'metacarpal bossing' appearance

(b) What are the treatment options for osteoarthritis of the hands?

Non-surgical:

- Physiotherapy may help to maintain functional ability, and especially with thumb involvement, splints may also be used
- Pain relief (using analgesic ladder – Case 118): paracetamol, aspirin or other non-steroidal anti-inflammatory drugs for symptomatic relief

Surgical:

- Joint arthrodesis, and in the case of thumb CMCJ involvement, trapeziectomy can be performed with tendinous interpositional graft (from flexor carpi radialis)
- Arthroplasty (with the Swanson silicone trapezium implant) has largely been abandoned due to the problems of dislocation and silicone-induced synovitis
- Heberdens and Bouchards nodes rarely require surgical management, but sometimes an arthrodesis is required if the joint becomes unstable or very painful

> *William Heberden (1710–1801)* also described angina, chicken pox and night blindness. 'Heberden Disease' is another name for angina pectoris. He was physician to George III and attended to Dr Johnson during his last illness.
> *C.J. Bouchard (1837–1925).* French physician who was also one of the initial physicians to describe spider naevi.

FURTHER READING

van Cappelle H G, Deutman R, van Horn J R (2001) Use of the Swanson silicone trapezium implant for treatment of primary osteoarthritis: long-term results. *J Bone Joint Surg Am* **83A**(7): 999–1004

Barron O A, Glickel S Z, Eaton R G (2000) Basal joint arthritis of the thumb. *J Am Acad Orthop Surg* **8**(5): 314–23

http://www.dynomed.com/encyclopedia/encyclopedia/arthritis/PIP-DIP_Osteoarthritis.html – information for patients

CASE 82   ULNAR NERVE LESIONS   * * *

INSTRUCTION

'Examine this gentleman's hands.'

APPROACH

Within surgical short cases the likely reason for weakness of the hand will be a specific neurological lesion of the median, ulnar or radial nerves. Beginning with the Top Tips (*see* Case 79) will allow the candidate to get swiftly to the diagnosis without wasting time.

Expose to elbows and ask the patient to place his hands palm upwards on a pillow (if available).

VITAL POINTS

Inspect

- Note the claw hand appearance, with paralysis of lumbricals and interossei, and unopposed action of the long flexors and extensors, causing flexed, deformed little and ring fingers (see difference between high and low lesions below)
- Examine the palm, noting the wasting of the hypothenar eminence (all muscles here are supplied by the ulnar nerve) (Fig. 32)

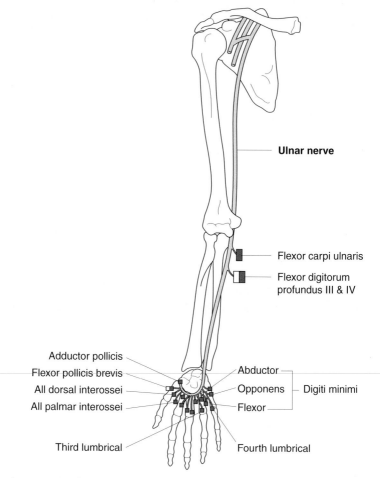

Ulnar nerve

Flexor carpi ulnaris

Flexor digitorum
profundus III & IV

Adductor pollicis
Flexor pollicis brevis
All dorsal interossei
All palmar interossei

Abductor ⎤
Opponens ⎬ Digiti minimi
Flexor ⎦

Third lumbrical

Fourth lumbrical

Fig. 32   Muscles supplied by the ulnar nerve.

- Ask the patient to turn his hands over and observe the guttering between the metacarpals as the interossei are wasted (best seen in the first dorsal webspace)

Sensory assessment

- Test the autonomous area (*see* Case 79) over the middle and distal phalanges of the little finger

Motor assessment

- Test the palmar interossei (which adduct the fingers) by asking the patient to hold a piece of paper between two fingers while you attempt to pull it away – you have now tested the autonomous motor supply (*see* Case 79)

- Continue to test the dorsal interossei (which abduct the fingers) by asking the patient to spread his fingers and prevent you from pushing them together
- Assess for weakness of flexor digitorum profundus to the ring and little fingers (*see* Case 88 – trigger finger)

Special tests

- Froment's sign – this test is based on the fact that adductor pollicis is supplied by the ulnar nerve, and if there is an ulnar nerve palsy, the only way to adduct the thumb is by using flexor pollicis longus to compensate (this muscle is supplied by the median nerve). Ask the patient to hold a piece of paper between the thumb and radial aspect of the index finger and as you pull this piece of paper away from the patient, observe the thumb – you will see the distal phalanx flex if the patient is using flexor pollicis longus to hold the piece of paper
- Elbow flexion test – with the elbow fully flexed, the patient will complain of numbness and tingling in the ring and little fingers, often within one minute – this test may be quite uncomfortable for the patient, and therefore you are better off describing it first to the examiner

---

TOP TIP
When examining the peripheral nerves of the upper limb begin at the hand and move proximally. Continue examining one nerve in its entirety before moving onto the next nerve, by which time the examiner will usually have stopped you. This allows a precise definition of the anatomical location of the nerve lesion described.

Finish your examination here

Completion

Tell the examiner you would examine the neck and all the other peripheral nerves of the affected limb.

QUESTIONS

(a) What causes do you know of ulnar nerve palsies?

The causes can be divided up according to broad aetiological categories:

- Anatomical – cubital tunnel syndrome at the elbow (due to repeated elbow flexion leading to traction injury +/– recurrent subluxation of the nerve within the tunnel)
- Trauma – anywhere along the course of the nerve, e.g. supracondylar fractures and dislocations of the elbow (also late sequelae of trauma can lead to ulnar nerve palsy, e.g. cubitus valgus deformity at the elbow)
- Degenerative arthritis – with compressing proliferative synovitis and osteophytes, or loose bodies
- Rare causes – compression from tight fascia or ligaments, tumour masses, aneurysms, vascular thromboses, or anomalous muscles (e.g. anconeus epitrochlearis)

(b) How do you clinically differentiate between a high and a low ulnar nerve lesion?

Low lesions (below elbow):

- More marked clawing as flexor digitorum profundus to ring and little fingers is still functioning

High lesions (above elbow):

- Paralysis of flexor digitorum profundus to ring and little fingers leads to less marked clawing of these fingers as the flexion component the clawing is less prominent – this is known as the 'ulnar paradox'
- Decreased sensation over ulnar border of the hand
- Otherwise as for low lesion

ADVANCED QUESTIONS

(a) How do you treat ulnar nerve palsies?

Non-surgical – for patients with mild, intermittent symptoms and no significant neurological deficits – avoid repetitive flexion-extension motions and prolonged elbow flexion, and use of night splintage with the elbow in extension

Surgical – for patients with persistent, significant symptoms or neurological deficit, surgical options include:

- Ulnar nerve decompression (decompression of the roof of the cubital tunnel at the elbow)
- Ulnar nerve anterior transposition +/– subcutaneous or submuscular transposition
- Medial epicondylectomy

Jules Froment (1878–1946). Neurologist and Professor of Clinical Medicine, Lyons, France.

FURTHER READING

Posner MA (2000) Compressive neuropathies of the ulnar nerve at the elbow and wrist. *Instr Course Lect* **49**: 305–17

| CASE 83 | HALLUX VALGUS *** |

INSTRUCTION

'Examine this lady's feet.'

APPROACH

Expose both ankles and feet and begin by describing any obvious deformities. You should position yourself either sitting on a chair facing the patient or kneeling on the ground opposite her.

VITAL POINTS

Look

- Unilateral or bilateral?
- Estimate degree of valgus of the big toe
- Is there rotation of the big toe (nail faces medially)?
- Is there a bunion present? – a bunion is a prominence of the medial aspect of the first metatarsal head with or without an overlying bursa
- Are there visible signs of inflammation of the bursa, e.g. erythema?
- Is there a hammered or retracted second toe (*see* Case 84)?
- Look at the soles of the feet – are there any callosities present?

Feel

- Is there any inflammation of the bunion, e.g. warmth, tenderness?
- Localize any areas of tenderness, e.g. osteoarthritis of the first metatarsophalangeal joint (MTPJ)

Move

- Assess range of movement of the first MTPJ, including noting the presence of any hypermobility (indicating instability)

Finish your examination here

Completion

Say that you would like to:

- Assess the range of motion of the other toe joints
- Watch the patient walk (gait) – this allows inspection of the heel and ankle from the back, again noting any gross deformities
- Examine her shoes – abnormalities of weightbearing will be reflected in the pattern of wear
- Ask her questions to assess the effect of the condition on her life

QUESTIONS

(a) Name one investigation you would perform in order to further assess the condition?

Plain weightbearing X-rays in order to assess:

- Degree of valgus deformity
- First/second intermetatarsal angle (IMA) and distal metatarsal articular angle (DMAA) (Fig. 33)
- Presence of osteoarthritis of the first MTPJ

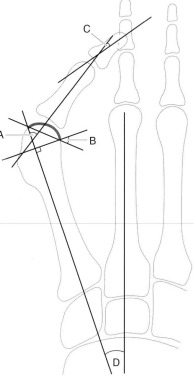

Fig. 33   Important radiological angles in hallux valgus. A = hallux valgus angle; B = distal metatarsal articulation angle; C = interphalangeal angle; D = inter-metatarsal angle.

(b) What do you know of the aetiology of hallux valgus?

- Essentially unknown
- Strong familial trait
- Increased incidence in people who wear enclosed footwear – rarely seen in those who have never worn shoes
- Associated with rheumatoid arthritis
- Secondary to metatarsus primus varus, which itself may be congenital or secondary to loss of muscle tone with age

(c) What treatment options are available in hallux valgus?

Non-surgical:

- Appropriate footwear, e.g. wide shoe with soft upper, wide toe box and protective padding over prominences (the surgeon should follow-up the patient after a couple of months in order to examine the footwear and note wear patterns)
- Physiotherapy

Surgical:

Several options are available, depending on the wishes of the patient, her level of activity and the state of her peripheral vascular system. These include:

- Bunionectomy
- First metatarsal realignment osteotomy
- Excision arthroplasty (Keller's procedure) – essentially a proximal hemiphalangectomy
- Fusion – for degenerative joint disease

ADVANCED QUESTION

(a) How would you decide which surgical techniques to use in a specific patient?

If the examiner moves you on to specific surgical options, a rough outline of treatment can be given, although decisions are tailored to the individual.

Arthritic joint:

- In active patient – first MTP arthrodesis or prosthetic arthroplasty
- Low-demand elderly patient – Keller's procedure (becoming less popular)

Non-arthritic joint:

- IMA < 15° – e.g. Chevron osteotomy
- IMA > 15° – e.g. scarf osteotomy

> *Colonel William Keller (1874–1959).* Director of Professional Services of the American Expeditionary Forces during World War I. He first devised the procedure in Manila during the Philippine War.

FURTHER READING

Ferrari J, Higgins J P, Williams R L (2000) Interventions for treating hallux valgus (abductovalgus) and bunions. Cochrane Database Syst Rev 2: CD000964

Coughlin M J (1997) Hallux valgus. *Instr Course Lect* **46**: 357–91

http://www.rad.washington.edu/anatomy/modules/HalluxValgus/HalluxValgus.html – good diagrams explaining how to interpret radiological features of hallux valgus

http://www.boa.ac.uk/bofss/halluxvalgus.htm – information for patients

★★★ HAMMER TOES CASE 84

INSTRUCTION

'Examine this lady's right foot'.

APPROACH

Expose both ankles and feet by removing socks and shoes, and begin by describing any obvious deformities

VITAL POINTS

Look

- Affects the lesser toes, most commonly the second toe
- May be associated with hallux valgus
- Flexion deformity at the proximal interphalangeal joint (PIPJ) of the involved toe(s) – this is the major deformity to note
- The distal interphalangeal joint (DIPJ) can be in any position, but extension is most common (Fig. 34)

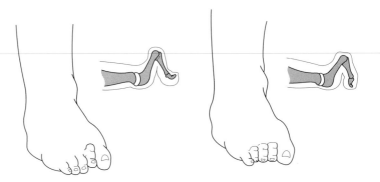

Fig. 34 Hammer toe (left) and claw toe (right).

- Neutral or extension at the metatarsophalangeal joint (MTPJ), although hammer toes deformities are primarily confined to the interphalangeal joints (compared with claw toes – *see* Case 86)
- Note any associated callosities

Feel

- Any tenderness of the affected toe(s)

Move

- Note whether deformity is fixed or mobile

Finish your examination here

Completion

Say that you would like to:

- Watch the patient walk
- Examine her shoes
- Ask her questions to assess the effect of the condition on her life

QUESTIONS

(a) What is the aetiology of hammer toes?

- Imbalance between intrinsic (lumbricals and interossei) and extrinsic (long flexors and extensors) muscles of the lesser toes
- More common in:
  - females than males
  - the elderly
  - patients with rheumatoid arthritis

(b) How would you treat this lady's condition?

Non-surgical:

- Appropriate footwear, e.g. high, wide toeboxes and semirigid longitudinal arch supports with metatarsal pads to evenly distribute plantar pressure

Surgical:

- Mobile deformity – consider flexor-to-extensor tendon transfer (split flexor digitorum longus transfer to the extensor hood – Girdlestone–Taylor procedure)
- Fixed deformity – consider:
  - resection of the proximal phalangeal head and neck with possible flexor and extensor release
  - proximal phalangectomy
  - PIPJ arthrodesis
- Painful callosities – consider terminal phalangectomy

Gathorne Robert Girdlestone (1881–1950). First Professor of Orthopaedic Surgery in Britain (at Oxford).

FURTHER READING

Harmonson J K, Harkless L B (1996) Operative procedures for the correction of hammertoe, claw toe, and mallet toe: a literature review. *Clin Podiatr Med Surg* **13**(2): 211–20

http://www.foot.com/html/hammer_toe.html – information for patients

INSTRUCTION

'Have a look at this lady's right foot.'

APPROACH

Expose both ankles and feet by removing socks and shoes, and begin by describing any obvious deformities.

VITAL POINTS

Look

- Affects the lesser toes, commonly the second toe
- Flexion deformity at the distal interphalangeal joint (DIPJ) of the involved toe(s)
- No proximal interphalangeal joint (PIPJ) or metatarsophalangeal joint (MTPJ) involvement
- Note any associated callosities

Feel

- Any tenderness of the affected toe(s)

Move

- Note whether deformity is fixed or mobile

Finish your examination here

Completion

Say that you would like to:

- Watch the patient walk
- Examine her shoes
- Ask her questions to assess the effect of the condition on her life

QUESTIONS

(a) What is the aetiology of mallet toes?

- As with hammer toes, imbalance between intrinsic (lumbricals and interossei) and extrinsic (long flexors and extensors) muscles of the lesser toes
- More common in females than males, the elderly and patients with rheumatoid arthritis and diabetics with peripheral neuropathy

(b) How would you treat this lady's condition?

Non-surgical:

- Appropriate footwear – usually unhelpful

Surgical:

- Mobile deformity – consider flexor digitorum longus tenotomy (if extensor digitorum longus tendon intact)
- Fixed deformity – consider:
  - flexor tenotomy with resection of the middle phalangeal head and neck
  - fusion of the DIPJ
  - amputation of distal half of distal phalanx to include nail and matrix

FURTHER READING

Harmonson J K, Harkless L B (1996) Operative procedures for the correction of hammertoe, claw toe, and mallet toe: a literature review. *Clin Podiatr Med Surg* **13**(2): 211–20.

CASE 86   **CLAW TOES**   ★ ★ ★

INSTRUCTION

'Examine this lady's right foot.'

APPROACH

Expose both ankles and feet (by removing socks and shoes) and begin by describing any obvious deformities.

VITAL POINTS

Look

- Affects the lesser toes – frequently all four involved
- May be bilateral
- Flexion deformity at the proximal interphalangeal joint (PIPJ) and distal interphalangeal joint (DIPJ) (*see* Fig. 34)
- Involves the metatarsophalangeal joint (MTPJ) – note MTPJ hyperextension
- Note any associated callosities – plantar to the metatarsal heads and dorsal to the PIPJs

Feel

- Any tenderness of the affected toe(s)

Move

- Note whether deformity is fixed or mobile

Finish your examination here

Completion

Say that you would like to:

- Watch the patient walk
- Examine her shoes
- Ask her questions to assess the effect of the condition on her life

QUESTIONS

(a) What is the aetiology of claw toes?

- As with hammer and mallet toes, imbalance between intrinsic (lumbricals and interossei) and extrinsic (long flexors and extensors) muscles of the lesser toes
- More common in females than males, the elderly and patients with rheumatoid arthritis
- May be secondary to neurological disorders such as peripheral neuropathy (diabetes, Charcot–Marie–Tooth disease), lower motor neurone disease (poliomyelitis) and upper motor neurone disease (cerebral palsy, multiple sclerosis, stroke)

(b) How would you treat this lady's condition?

Non-surgical:

- Appropriate footwear, e.g. high, wide toeboxes and semirigid longitudinal arch supports with metatarsal pads to evenly distribute plantar pressure

Surgical:

- Mobile deformity – consider flexor-to-extensor tendon transfer (*see* hammer toes, Case 84)
- Fixed deformity – consider:
  - resection of the proximal phalangeal head and neck with possible flexor and extensor release
  - extensor tenotomy for contractures of the MTPJ
  - resection of the metatarsal heads of the lesser toes

Jean-Martin Charcot (1825–1893). See Charcot's joints (Case 103).
Pierre Marie (1853–1940). Professor of Pathological Anatomy and Clinical Neurology, Salpetriere Hospital, Paris.
Howard Henry Tooth (1856–1926). English physician and neurologist.
Charcot-Marie-Tooth syndrome (peroneal muscular atrophy) presents in puberty or early adult life and causes progressive weakness of the peroneal muscles, the foot and toe dorsiflexors, the plantar flexors and the intrinsic muscles of the foot, leading to claw toes, and varus and cavus deformities of the forefoot and hindfoot. It may also affect the median and ulnar nerves.

FURTHER READING

Harmonson J K, Harkless L B (1996) Operative procedures for the correction of hammertoe, claw toe, and mallet toe: a literature review. *Clin Podiatr Med Surg* **13**(2): 211–20.

CASE 87   **MALLET FINGER**   ★★★

INSTRUCTION

'Examine this gentleman's hand.'

APPROACH

Expose the patient as for any hand examination, asking him to place his hands palms upwards on a white pillow.

VITAL POINTS

Look

- Note the flexion deformity of the distal phalanx of one or more of the fingers

Move

- Test for active movement of the finger – the terminal phalanx cannot be actively extended
- On passive movement of the joint the digit can be moved back into the normal position (unless chronic)

Finish your examination here

QUESTIONS

(a) What is the aetiology of mallet finger?

There has been damage (usually division) of the extensor tendon to the terminal phalanx of the finger involved. This may occur if a flake of bone is avulsed from the base of the distal phalanx (thus the term baseball finger, as this avulsion may occur in catching a ball).

Interestingly, note that in rheumatoid arthritis, rupture of the central slip of the extensor tendon more proximally leads to the classic Boutonniere's deformity (*see* Case 80).

(b) How is mallet finger managed when presenting acutely?

The finger should be X-rayed to exclude a fracture. The finger should be splinted for 6 weeks with the distal interphalangeal joint in extension in a mallet splint to allow reattachment of the tendon. If the avulsed flake of bone is greater than a third of the width of the joint space on the lateral X-ray, it should be repositioned with a fine Kirschner (K) wire or other internal fixation device.

> *Martin Kirschner (1879–1942).* A pupil of Trendelenburg who became Professor of Surgery in Heidelberg, Germany.

FURTHER READING

Perron A D, Brady W J, Keats T E, Hersh R E (2001) Orthopedic pitfalls in the emergency department: closed tendon injuries of the hand. *Am J Emerg Med* **19**(1): 76–80

Burke F (1988) Mallet finger. *Br J Hand Surg* **13**(2): 115–7

http://www.eatonhand.com/clf/clf002.htm – information for patients

---

** ** TRIGGER FINGER   CASE 88

INSTRUCTION

'Examine this gentleman's hand.'

APPROACH

Expose the patient as for any hand examination, asking him to place his hands palms upwards on a white pillow.

VITAL POINTS

Look

Note flexion of one or more of the fingers. However, the finger does not necessarily have to be fixed in flexion the whole time for it to be triggering. Trigger finger most frequently affects the middle or ring fingers.

Feel

Ask the patient if there is any pain and then palpate carefully over the palm proximal to the finger involved, as there may be a small nodule overlying the flexor tendon sheath as it enters the digit. The nodule is usually approximately at the level of the proximal transverse palmar crease.

Move

Test for *active* movement of the finger and note that on gentle forced extension of the finger, there may be a characteristic snap as the distal finger passes the obstruction.

TOP TIP – Examination of the flexor tendons of the hand

- Place the patient's hand flat on a hard surface with the palms facing upwards
- Flexor digitorum profunda tendon is tested by active flexion of the distal interphalangeal joint, with the PIPJ fixed in full extension
- Flexor digitorum superficialis tendon is tested by active flexion of the PIPJ when the examiner fixes the other fingers in full extension

---

Finish your examination here

QUESTIONS

(a) What is the aetiology of trigger finger?

Trigger finger is caused by fibrosis and thickening of the flexor tendon sheath as the tendon enters the digit. They may be idiopathic, or may follow trauma or some unusual activity. Occasionally they can be congenital and present in children. The other name for this condition is stenosing tenovaginitis. A similar triggering may occur in rheumatoid arthritis, when other signs of rheumatoid arthritis of the hands would be expected.

(b) How is trigger finger treated?

If a nodule is present over the flexor tendon sheath then a steroid injection may be of benefit but often a tendon release, by incising the sheath, is required.

FURTHER READING

Turowski G A, Zdankiewicz P D, Thomson J G (1997) The results of surgical treatment of trigger finger. *Am J Hand Surg* **22**(1): 145–9

** INGROWING TOENAIL　　　　　　CASE 89

INSTRUCTION

'Look at this gentleman's feet and tell me what you would do about his problem.'

APPROACH

Expose both feet for comparison.

VITAL POINTS

Inspect

- Most commonly affects the lateral aspect of the great toenail
- Lateral aspect of the nail seen to be digging into the substance of the toe
- Look for signs of inflammation such as swelling and erythema
- Look for evidence of serous or purulent discharge

Finish your examination here

> TOP TIP
> If this diagnosis is obvious, tell the examiner immediately what is wrong and move on to discuss the treatment options.

QUESTIONS

(a) What treatments are available for ingrowing toenails?

Non-surgical: good nail care, with the help of a chiropodist, trimming nail transversely, using cotton wool packs to lift up the nail and keeping the foot clean and dry.

Surgical options include:

- Simple nail avulsion
  - best treatment for acutely infected toes as nail-bed treatment carries the risk of osteomyelitis in the presence of infection; recurrence and regrowth are common
  - when combined with the use of phenol, recurrence is less common, but this increases the risk of postoperative infection
- Wedge excision
  - excision of the involved aspect (lateral or medial) of the nail and nail-bed with a wedge of the nail fold down to the periosteum of the phalanx distal to the joint
- Zadek's procedure
  - total excision of the nailbed including the germinal matrix

(b) What are the complications of ingrowing toenail surgery?

- Wound infection
- Regrowth
- Osteomyelitis and septic arthritis

FURTHER READING

Rounding C, Hulm S (2000) Surgical treatments for ingrowing toenails. *Cochrane Database Syst Rev* (2): CD001541

Murray WR (1989) Management of ingrowing toenail. *Br J Surg* **76**(9): 883–4

http://www.boa.ac.uk/bofss/igtnfor.htm – information for patients

---

CASE 90	INTERNAL DERANGEMENT OF THE KNEE	**

INSTRUCTION

'Examine this gentleman's right knee.'

APPROACH

Proceed with the routine knee examination (*see* Case 77)

VITAL POINTS

Inspect standing (front and back)

- Scars – look particularly for:
  - arthroscopic portal scars – anteromedial and anterolateral scars found in the triangle between the patella tendon, tibial plateau and femoral condyle
  - meniscectomy scars – 5 cm scar over anteromedial aspect of knee joint for open medial meniscectomy and 5.5 cm scar over anterolateral aspect of knee for open lateral meniscectomy
- Valgus or varus deformity of the knee – may be secondary to an old meniscectomy resulting in secondary osteoarthritis

Gait

- Antalgic – if the knee is painful, e.g. secondary to a meniscal tear or recent injury

Measure

- Quadriceps wasting may be demonstrated (*see* Case 77)

Feel (lying supine)

- Tenderness
  - medial joint line – indicates medial meniscal tear
  - lateral joint line – indicates lateral meniscal tear
- Effusion – may be a sympathetic effusion secondary to a cruciate ligament or meniscal injury

Move

- Block to extension = locked knee (indicates meniscal or cruciate ligament injury)

Special tests

- Cruciate ligaments
  - posterior sag – posterior cruciate ligament (PCL) injury
  - anterior drawer – anterior cruciate ligament (ACL) injury
  - posterior drawer – PCL injury
  - positive Lachman's test (most sensitive) – ACL injury
- Collateral ligaments
  - medial joint line opens up on stress testing – medial collateral ligament (MCL) injury
  - lateral joint line opens up on stress testing – lateral collateral ligament (LCL) injury
- Menisci
  - positive McMurray's test – medial or lateral meniscal tear

Finish your examination here

Completion

Say that you would like to:

- Examine the hip and ankle (the joint above and below the knee joint)
- Assess the neurovascular status of the limb
- Ask the patient some questions to ascertain how much the problem affects his life, e.g. work, sports, etc

QUESTIONS

(a) Cruciate ligament injuries are one cause of haemarthrosis of the knee. What other causes can you think of?

- Primary spontaneous haemarthrosis
  - occurs without trauma
  - may be secondary to disorders of coagulation or vascular malformations
- Secondary haemarthrosis
  - secondary to trauma
  - 80% are due to ACL injury
  - 10% are secondary to patellar dislocation

– 10% follow tears in the peripheral third of the menisci (where the meniscus is vascularised), capsular tears and osteochondral or osteophyte fractures

(b) What factors in the history point to an ACL injury?

- Most commonly associated with valgus/external rotation, hyperextension, deceleration and rotational movements
- Patient hears a 'pop' or feels something tear in > 50% of cases
- Inability to continue sport or activity
- Effusion (haemarthrosis) developing within 4–6 hours

(c) What are the problems associated with ACL rupture?

Abnormal knee movements occur leading to:

- Meniscal tears
- MCL injury
- Progressive premature osteoarthritis

(d) How do you treat a meniscal tear?

Treatment depends on age, chronicity of injury, activity requirements and location, type and length of tear, but there are options available.

Non-surgical – no intervention; treat symptomatically

Surgical:

- Arthroscopic or open
- Partial meniscectomy
- Meniscal repair
- Meniscal transplant (novel technique)

ADVANCED QUESTIONS

(a) What do you know of the anatomy of the menisci?

Medial meniscus:

- Semicircular
- Anterior horn attaches to the anterior intercondylar fascia of the tibia anterior to the ACL tibial insertion
- Posterior horn attaches posteriorly to the intercondylar fascia between the PCL tibial insertion and the posterior insertion of the lateral meniscus
- Bound to the joint capsule peripherally
- Bound to the femur and tibia at its midportion by the deep medial collateral ligament

Lateral meniscus:

- Nearly circular
- Covers a greater area of the tibial articular surface than the medial meniscus
- Anterior horn attaches to the tibial eminence behind the ACL tibial insertion

- Posterior horn attaches behind the tibial eminence anterior to the posterior edge of the medial meniscus
- Loosely attached to its respective tibial plateau by a capsular apron known as the coronary ligament

  Medial and lateral menisci are connected to each other anteriorly via the transverse ligament

(b) What do you know of the anatomy of the cruciate ligaments?

Anterior cruciate ligament:

- Intracapsular
- Originates from the medial aspect of the lateral femoral condyle
- Inserts into the anterolateral aspect of the medial tibial plateau
- Stops tibia moving forward (anteriorly) in relation to the femur (and also resists tibial rotation and varus-valgus angulation)
- Consists of two bundles, the anteromedial (tight in flexion and posterolateral (tight in extension) bands

Posterior cruciate ligament:

- Intraarticular but extrasynovial
- Broad origin forming a semicircle on the lateral aspect of the medial femoral condyle
- Inserts in a depression 1 cm inferior to the articular surface on the posterolateral aspect between the medial and lateral tibial plateaus
- Stops tibia moving backwards (posteriorly) in relation to the femur
- Consists of two functional components, the naterolateral group (tight in flexion) and the anteromedial group (tight in extension)

(c) How do you treat ACL ruptures?

Non-surgical – intensive physiotherapy:

- Re-education of quadriceps and hamstrings; note that the hamstrings restrict the amount of forward movement of the tibia in relation to the femur
- The results of physiotherapy can be predicted by Noyes' rule of thirds – a third will compensate and pursue normal recreational sports, a third will reduce sporting activities with avoidance of jumping and pivoting exercises, and a third will do poorly and develop instability with sporting and activities of daily living, thus needing early surgery

Surgical:

- Intraarticular reconstruction – commonly autologous hamstring tendon or bone-patellar tendon-bone graft
- Extraarticular reconstruction – e.g. MacIntosh tenodesis
- Combination of both the above

(d) What are the causes of a locked knee?

Causes can be classified by age. Causes in childhood include:

- Discoid meniscus
- Pathology in the hip
- Femoral condyle dysplasia

Adolescent causes are:

- Meniscal tear
- Cruciate ligament injury
- Osteochondritis dissecans
- Synovial chondromatosis

Adult:

- Meniscal tear
- Cruciate ligament injury
- Loose body
- Osteochondral fracture
- Synovial chondromatosis

Elderly:

- Meniscal tears
- Loose body
- Intraarticular tumour

FURTHER READING

Iobst C A, Stanitski C L (2000) Acute knee injuries. *Clin Sports Med* **19**(4): 621–35, vi

Bartlett R J, Clatworthy M G, Nguyen T N (2001) Graft selection in reconstruction of the anterior cruciate ligament. *J Bone Joint Surg (Br)* **83**(5): 625–34

Larson R V, Friedman M J (1996) Anterior cruciate ligament: injuries and treatment. *Instr Course Lect* **45**: 235–43

http://www.arthroscopy.com/sp05018.htm – pictorial explanation of anterior cruciate ligament reconstruction

** RADIAL NERVE LESIONS   **CASE 91**

INSTRUCTION

'This gentleman is complaining of weakness of his right hand. Have a look at his hands and tell me what you think the problem may be.'

APPROACH

Within surgical short cases the likely reason for weakness of the hand will be a specific neurological lesion, of the median, ulnar or radial nerves. Beginning with the Top Tips (*see* Case 79) will allow you to get swiftly to the diagnosis without wasting time.

Expose to elbows and ask the patient to place his hands palm upwards on a pillow (if available). To observe wrist drop, ask him to keep his hands out in front of him, palms downward.

VITAL POINTS

Inspect

- There is unlikely to be any wasting of the hand muscles but the hand is held with the wrist and fingers flexed (drop wrist)
- If the radial nerve has been damaged at the origin in the brachial plexus the whole arm is deformed (as in Erb's palsy, *see* Case 100)

Sensory assessment

- Note the loss of sensation over the 1st dorsal interosseus, which is on the dorsum of the hand between the thumb and index finger
- Test also for sensory loss over the dorsal aspect of the forearm

Motor assessment

- Begin with the metocarpophalangeal extensors (Top Tip Case 79) and note that extension is lost (Fig. 35)
- Fix the MCPJ extensors and demonstrate that extension at the PIPJ is preserved as the lumbricals and interossei are supplied by the median (lateral 2 lumbricals) and ulnar (rest of muscles) nerves
- Finally test triceps (extension of the elbow) to demonstrate weakness in high radial nerve lesions

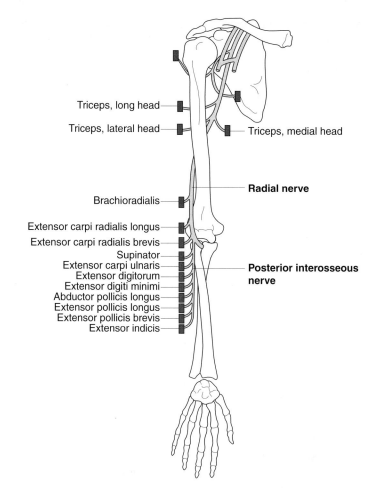

Triceps, long head

Triceps, lateral head

Triceps, medial head

Radial nerve

Brachioradialis

Extensor carpi radialis longus
Extensor carpi radialis brevis
Supinator
Extensor carpi ulnaris
Extensor digitorum
Extensor digiti minimi
Abductor pollicis longus
Extensor pollicis longus
Extensor pollicis brevis
Extensor indicis

Posterior interosseous nerve

Fig. 35   Muscles supplied by the radial nerve.

TOP TIP

When examining the peripheral nerves of the upper limb begin at the hand and move proximally. Continue examining one nerve in its entirety before moving onto the next nerve, by which time the examiner will usually have stopped you. This allows a precise definition of the anatomical location of the nerve lesion described.

Finish your examination here

Completion

Tell the examiner you would examine the neck and all the other peripheral nerves of the affected limb.

QUESTIONS

(a) What are the likely causes of a radial nerve lesion?

High lesions:

- Occur at the level of the brachial plexus, usually by crutches or Saturday night palsy (secondary to falling asleep with arm leaning over the top of a chair, thus compressing the radial nerve in the axilla – usually secondary to a state of alcoholic stupor!)
- This causes loss of extension of the elbow, wrist drop and loss of sensation over the 1st dorsal interosseus webspace

Middle lesions:

- Occur in the spiral groove of the humerus, usually as a result of a fracture of the middle third of the humerus, sometimes secondary to the use of a tourniquet
- In some instances the elbow is preserved, as the supply to the elbow leaves the main trunk of the nerve before it enters the groove

Low lesions:

- These occur at the elbow, due to local wounds, surgery or fracture/dislocations
- Only the posterior interosseus branch of the nerve is involved and sensation is preserved. The only lesion will be the loss of extension at the MCPJ

ADVANCED QUESTIONS

(a) What is Wartenberg's syndrome?

Compression of the sensory component of the radial nerve as it exits from under brachioradialis at the wrist. This is an unusual situation where an even more distal lesion can actually cause a sensory loss over the 1st dorsal interosseus.

FURTHER READING

Plate A M, Green S M (2000) Compressive radial neuropathies. *Instr Course Lect* **49**: 295–304

| CASE 92 | EXAMINATION OF THE SHOULDER | ** |

INSTRUCTION

'Examine this gentleman's right shoulder. He is complaining of difficulty in moving it.'

Note

The three most common pathologies that you may encounter in the exam are rotator cuff tears, impingement syndrome and frozen shoulder (adhesive capsulitis). The latter two are less common as they can be very painful.

APPROACH

You need to be able to see both shoulder joints – ask him to take off his shirt to adequately expose both upper limbs. If the patient is female, you would need to ask her to undress down to her bra to be able to see both shoulders (in which case you may wish to ask for a chaperone).

VITAL POINTS

Look (FROM FRONT AND BEHIND)

- Skin – scars, sinuses
- Symmetry – looking particularly for wasting of:
  - deltoid – loss of contour of shoulder
  - supraspinatus – look at the muscle bulk above the spine of the scapula from behind
  - infraspinatus – look at the muscle bulk below the spine of the scapula from behind
- Shape, looking particularly for:
  - prominent sternoclavicular joint (SCJ) – due to subluxation or osteoarthritis
  - clavicular deformity – due to old fracture
  - prominent acromioclavicular joint (ACJ) – due to subluxation

Feel

- Skin – increased temperature
- Bones and joints – systematically work your way laterally starting at the SCJ, feeling for tenderness:
  - SCJ
  - clavicle
  - ACJ
  - acromion
  - humeral head
  - greater tuberosity
  - coracoid

- Tendons:
  - long head of biceps – can be palpated for tenderness anteriorly in the bicipital groove as the shoulder is internally and externally rotated
  - supraspinatus – can be palpated just under the anterior edge of the acromion as the shoulder is held in extension

Move

Stand opposite the patient and ask him to imitate you in order to test active movements. Normal ranges of movement are:

- Forward flexion to 165° – 'Lift both your arms forwards'
- Abduction to 180° (of which the first 90° is glenohumeral, although scapulothoracic movement starts at 30–40° abduction) – 'Lift both your arms up to the side'
  - if there is difficulty initiating abduction or the humeral head rises up, consider rotator cuff tear
  - if there is a painful arc from 60–120°, think of rotator cuff tendinitis (also known as impingement syndrome) or a minor rotator cuff tear
  - if there is a painful arc from 140–180° i.e. a painful high arc, think of osteoarthritis of the ACJ
- External rotation to 60° (with the elbow flexed to 90° and tucked into the side of the body)
  - this movement is most commonly affected in frozen shoulder
- Internal rotation measured as thumb reaching mid-thoracic level (T6) – 'put your hand behind your back and reach up as far as you can'

You can then test the passive range of the same movements, but prevent scapulothoracic movement by anchoring the scapula (press firmly down on top of the shoulder with one hand).

This is followed by testing for power, particularly of:

- Deltoid – test abduction against resistance – an axillary nerve palsy can result in decreased deltoid power, with loss of sensation in the 'regimental badge' (British) area of skin of the shoulder
- Serratus anterior – pushing against a wall may demonstrate winging of the scapula secondary to a long thoracic nerve palsy (*see* Case 104)

TOP TIP

The mnemonic '**SITS**' can be used to remind you of the tendons of the rotator cuff:

Supraspinatus (abductor)
Infraspinatus (external rotator)
Teres minor (external rotator)
Subscapularis (internal rotator)

Special tests

You can test each muscle of the rotator cuff (see Mnemonic) individually for pain (in rotator cuff tendinitis) and weakness (in rotator cuff tears):

- Supraspinatus – resisted abduction with arm in maximum internal rotation with 20° abduction and 20° flexion – if torn, the patient cannot initiate abduction
- Infraspinatus/teres minor – resisted external rotation with elbow flexed to 90°
- Subscapularis – the most sensitive test is Gerber's lift-off test where the shoulder is internally rotated with the arm behind the back and the hand is resisted from being lifted off posteriorly; resisted internal rotation can be tested with the elbow flexed to 90°, but this does not isolate subscapularis

If you have time, you can also test specifically for biceps tendon pathology:

- Resisted elbow flexion with forearm in neutral rotation – biceps bulges if the long head is ruptured ('Popeye' bulge)
- Speed's test – resisted forward flexion of the shoulder with the elbow extended and the forearm supinated
- Yergason's test – resisted supination with the elbow flexed to 90°

Finish your examination here

Completion

Say that you would like to:

- Examine the neck (joint above) and elbow (joint below)
- Assess the neurovascular status of the limb
- Ask the patient some questions to assess how the condition affects his life

QUESTIONS

(a) What are the causes of a painful shoulder?

These can be divided up into:

- Tendon (rotator cuff) disorders:
  - tendinitis
  - rupture
  - frozen shoulder
- Joint disorders:
  - glenohumeral arthritis
  - acromioclavicular arthritis
- Referred pain:
  - cervical spondylosis
  - cardiac ischaemia
  - mediastinal pathology
- Instability:
  - dislocation
  - subluxation

- Bone lesions:
  - infection
  - neoplasms
- Nerve lesions
  - suprascapular nerve entrapment

(b) What is the aetiology of rotator cuff impingement?

- Repetitive rubbing of rotator cuff tendons under the coracoacromial arch (the coracoacromial ligament forms the roof of this arch and runs between the coracoid process anteriorly and the anterior third of the acromion posteriorly)
- The greatest amount of wear occurs in the 'impingement position' – abduction, slight flexion and internal rotation
- Site of impingement – 'critical area' of decreased vascularity in the supraspinatus tendon about 1 cm proximal to its insertion into the greater tuberosity
- Contributing factors to impingement:
  - bone – osteoarthritic thickening of ACJ; osteophytes anterior edge of acromion
  - tendon – rotator cuff swelling (in inflammatory disorders such as rheumatoid arthritis and gout)
  - bursa – subacromial bursitis (in inflammatory disorders as above)

(c) How do you treat impingement syndrome?

Non-surgical:

- Eliminate aggravating activity/avoid 'impingement position'
- Physiotherapy
- Short courses of analgesia, e.g. nonsteroidal anti-inflammatory drugs
- Subacromial corticosteroid injections for pain relief

Surgical:

- Open or arthroscopic subacromial decompression

(d) How do you treat rotator cuff tears?

Non-surgical:

- Physiotherapy to improve overall shoulder muscle strength

Surgical:

- Open or arthroscopic cuff repair (if amenable to repair) and subacromial decompression
- Open or arthroscopic cuff debridement (if not amenable to repair) and subacromial decompression

ADVANCED QUESTIONS

(a) What are the causes of a frozen shoulder?

Primary frozen shoulder (adhesive capsulitis):

- Often idiopathic
- Strong associations with diabetes and Dupuytren's contracture

- Global contracture of the shoulder joint, but maximally in the rotator interval area and around the coracohumeral ligament
- Histologically, the contracture is made of a dense collagen matrix, with numerous fibroblasts and myofibroblasts – this active fibroblast and myofibroblast proliferation is similar to the histology of Dupuytren's contracture (*see* Case 78)
- Recently, there has been accumulating evidence that the frozen shoulder may remain 'frozen' due to slow remodelling as a result of high levels of tissue inhibitors of metalloproteinases (TIMPSs), which inhibit matrix metalloproteinases (MMPs)

Secondary frozen shoulder:

- Intrinsic causes:
  - chronic rotator cuff injuries
  - post-traumatic scarring following fractures around the shoulder, e.g. surgical neck or tuberosity fractures
- Extrinsic causes – painful disorders leading to decreased movements of the shoulder:
  - referred pain from cervical radiculopathy
  - post-hand, wrist or elbow surgery
  - post-breast surgery (especially when axillary node dissection has been performed)
  - post-myocardial infarct

(b) How do you treat a frozen shoulder?

Non-surgical:

- Pain relief – analgesic ladder (*see* Case 118), interscalene blocks
- Physiotherapy – especially pendulum exercises
- Manipulation under anaesthesia and steroid/local anaesthetic injections – once acute pain has settled

Surgical:

- Surgery has an ill-defined role
- Reserved for prolonged and disabling restriction
- Open or arthroscopic rotator interval, coracohumeral ligament release and excision of the coracoacromial ligament

FURTHER READING

McConville O R, Iannotti J P (1999) Partial-thickness tears of the rotator cuff: evaluation and management. *J Am Acad Orthop Surg* **7**(1): 32–43

Bunker T D (1997) Frozen shoulder: unravelling the enigma. *Ann R Coll Surg Engl* **79**(3): 210–3

Morrison D S, Greenbaum B S, Einhorn A (2000) Shoulder impingement. *Orthop Clin North Am* **31**(2): 285–93

http://orthoinfo.aaos.org/brochure/thr_report.cfm?Thread_ID=43&topcategory= Shoulder – patient information website on shoulder pain

http://www.nismat.org/orthocor/exam/shoulder.html – how to examine the
   shoulder with excellent anatomical models showing the various joints and
   tendons around the shoulder girdle and clinical photographs

http://www.med.und.nodak.edu/depts/fpc/aaron/examt.htm – another website on
   how to examine the shoulder, but with Quicktime movie files to demonstrate
   the various techniques

** GAIT   CASE 93

INSTRUCTION

'This gentleman has an abnormal gait. Watch him walk and tell me what you make
of it.'

APPROACH

This is a potentially difficult case as often the different abnormal gaits can be problematic to distinguish.

   Expose the patient's lower limb keeping his underwear on but ask him to remove
his socks and shoes.

VITAL POINTS

Inspect

- Ask the patient to walk towards a given point at the other side of the room and
  then back towards you
- Note if he has difficulty in initiating movement or other signs of Parkinson's
  disease
- Look to see if the patient grimaces as if with pain (do they have an antalgic gait?)

Finish your examination here

Completion

Tell the examiner you would:
- Examine the back and hip joints, including performing a Trendelenburg test
  (*see* Case 76)
- Measure the leg lengths (in short leg gait) (*see* Case 76)
- Examine the lower limb neurology, looking specifically for footdrop (see below)

QUESTIONS

(a) What are the phases of gait?

Four phases make up the gait:

- Heel strike
- Stance, when foot is on the ground and the centre of gravity of the body moves
  forward

- Toe off, as the foot begins to lift off the ground from the heel forward
- Swing, as the foot moves forward while the contralateral foot supports the weight of the body

(b) What are the common abnormalities of gait?

Table 26 summarizes the various abnormalities you would be expected to know about.

Table 26

Type of gait	Description	Reason for abnormality
Antalgic	Decreased stance and increased swing phase	Pain
Trendelenburg (see Case 76)	Hip dips instead of rising when foot is lifted off floor, shoulders also lurch to opposite side	Abductor weakness
Parkinsonian	Small shuffling steps (= festinant gait)	Parkinson's disease
Broad based	Reels, lurches to one side	Cerebellar lesions
Short leg	Ipsilateral hip drops when weight is on short leg	Previous fracture or congenital shortening
High stepping	Foot lands flat or on ball instead of on heel, with foot 'slapping' to the ground	Foot drop – inability to dorsiflex the foot secondary to damage to L5 (which supplies extensor hallucis longus, extensor digitorum longus and tibialis anterior) – this is most commonly due to common peroneal nerve palsy (e.g. trauma to fibular head, tight casts) or sciatic nerve palsy (e.g. gunshot wounds, posterior hip dislocations, posterior approach during surgery to the hip joint)
Spastic	Jerky, feet in equinus, hips adducted ('scissoring')	Likely to be an upper motor neurone cause such as cord compression, multiple sclerosis or cerebral palsy

FURTHER READING

Devinney S, Prieskorn D (2000) Neuromuscular examination of the foot and ankle. *Foot Ankle Clin* **5**(2): 213–33

** OSTEOCHONDROMA   CASE 94

INSTRUCTION

'Examine this lump and tell me your diagnosis.'

APPROACH

Expose the relevant area – note that osteochondromas are adjacent to the epiphyseal line in the diaphyseal side of the bone and that they are most commonly found around the knee joint (lower end of the femur or upper end of the tibia).

Examine as for lumps (Case 1).

VITAL POINTS

Inspect

- Hemispherical lump
- Solitary or multiple (the latter may be part of hereditary multiple exostoses)

Palpate

- Smooth surface
- Narrow base
- Osteochondromas point away from the joint
- May be bony-hard in consistency or soft if there is an overlying bursa
- Move the adjacent joint while palpating the lump and assess the relationship with adjacent muscle and tendons, and degree of interference with joint movement

QUESTIONS

(a) What is an osteochondroma?

- Lump of cancellous bone with a covering of cortical bone and a cartilaginous cap
- They originate from the separation of small pieces of metaphyseal cartilage from the main cartilaginous epiphyseal plate. These small pieces escape remodelling and carry on growing and ossifying
- Usually start to grow in adolescence

ADVANCED QUESTIONS

(a) What is diaphyseal aclasis?

- An autosomal dominant condition, characterized by multiple osteochondromas particularly in the limb bones

- All bones that ossify in cartilage can be affected except the spine and skull
- It is thought to be a failure of growth-plate modelling
- There is a small incidence of sarcomatous change, particularly if subjected to trauma

(b) What is the surgical treatment?

The osteochondroma should be excised if symptomatic (such as pressure symptoms, cosmesis) or if it increases in size or becomes more painful (suspicion of malignancy)

FURTHER READING

Miller S L, Hoffer F A (2001) Malignant and benign bone tumors. *Radiol Clin North Am* **39**(4): 673–99

| CASE 95 | POPLITEAL FOSSA SWELLINGS | ✱✱ |

INSTRUCTION

'Examine this gentleman's right knee.'

APPROACH

Approach as for knee examination (*see* Case 77).

VITAL POINTS

You should aim to elicit features of a lump (*see* Case 1) – the vital points are outlined below.

Look from behind and from the side (with the patient standing)

- Visible swelling in the popliteal fossa (proceed with the following routine, leaving 'gait' and 'measure' until you have fully described this swelling)
- Skin involvement – sebaceous cyst

Palpate from behind

- Pulsatile (swelling overlying popliteal artery) or expansile (popliteal artery aneurysm)
- Fluctuant (cystic swelling)
- Compressible (saphena varix of the saphenopopliteal junction)
- Transilluminable (cystic swelling)

Finish your examination here

Completion

Say you would like to:

- Continue with the rest of the knee examination (the examiner may allow you to proceed if there are further signs to elicit, e.g. osteoarthritis of the knee)
- Perform a neurological and peripheral vascular examination, including the peripheral pulses
- Examine the joint above (the hip) and the joint below (the ankle)

QUESTIONS

(a) What is your differential diagnosis?

- Skin and subcutaneous tissues – lipoma (*see* Case 2), sebaceous cyst (*see* Case 3)
- Artery – popliteal artery aneurysm (*see* Case 117)
- Vein – saphena varix (at the saphenopopliteal junction, *see* Case 109), deep vein thrombosis
- Nerve – neuroma (e.g. tibial nerve)
- Enlarged bursae, e.g. associated with semimembranosus and medial head of gastrocnemius medially and with popliteus and lateral head of gastrocnemius laterally (Fig. 36)
- Cysts – Baker's cyst (associated with degenerative changes in the knee joint) and popliteal cyst (enlargement of the popliteal bursa but the knee joint is normal)

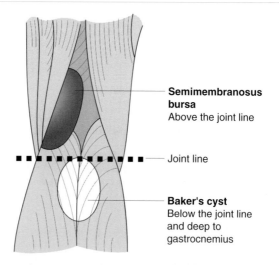

Semimembranosus bursa
Above the joint line

Joint line

Baker's cyst
Below the joint line and deep to gastrocnemius

Fig. 36 Anatomical difference between a semimembranosus bursa and a Baker's cyst.

(b) What is a Baker's cyst?

- Described by Baker as a posterior herniation of the capsule of the knee joint
- Leads to escape of synovial fluid into one of the posterior bursae, stiffness and knee swelling
- Often associated with degenerative knee joint disease
- Diagnosis is confirmed by ultrasound examination – identification of fluid between the semimembranosus and medial gastrocnemius tendons in communication with a posterior knee cyst indicates Baker's cyst with 100% accuracy
- Aspiration is possible, although recurrence is common
- Important to rule out deep vein thrombosis, but the two can co-exist

(c) What is a popliteal cyst?

- Usually located on the medial side of popliteal fossa, just distal to the flexion crease of the knee, under the medial head of gastrocnemius
- Found in children and young adults (in adults, may be associated with pathology in the knee)
- Twice as common in boys compared with girls
- Usually unilateral
- Becomes more prominent when knee extended and disappears in flexion
- Firm and can be transilluminated
- If the cyst is not found in the medial part of the popliteal fossa or has a solid component (on ultrasound), rule out tumour with a CT or MRI scan
- Cysts can either be aspirated and sent for cytology if the patient (or the child's parents) are concerned, or surgically excised
- Although spontaneous remission is not to be expected in all cases, asymptomatic popliteal cysts in children can be treated non-surgically with good results

ADVANCED QUESTIONS

(a) What are the boundaries of the popliteal fossa?

- Superomedial – semimembranosus and semitendinosus tendons
- Superolateral – biceps tendon
- Inferomedial – medial head of gastrocnemius
- Inferolateral – lateral head of gastrocnemius
- Roof – fascia lata
- Floor – (from proximal to distal) popliteal surface of the femur, capsule of the knee joint and popliteus muscle covered by its fascia

---

William Morrant Baker (1839–1896). English Surgeon, St Bartholomew's Hospital, London. Private assistant to Sir James Paget.

FURTHER READING

Ward E E, Jacobson J A, Fessell D P, Hayes C W, van Holsbeeck M (2001) Sonographic detection of Baker's cysts: comparison with MR imaging. *AJR Am J Roentgenol* **176**(2): 373–80

Van Rhijn L W, Jansen E J, Pruijs H E (2000) Long-term follow-up of conservatively treated popliteal cysts in children. *J Pediatr Orthop B* **9**(1): 62–4

** HALLUX RIGIDUS   CASE 96

INSTRUCTION

'Examine this gentleman's right foot.'

APPROACH

Expose both ankles and feet and begin by describing any obvious deformities.

VITAL POINTS

Look (and ask)

- Likely to be unremarkable – if you notice no abnormalities on initial inspection, ask the gentleman where exactly the problem is in order to focus your examination on the big toe (this will stop you wasting time examining all the joints of the foot)
- Note that he is likely to be complaining of pain in the right big toe on weightbearing, particularly during the push-off phase of gait

Feel

- First metatarsophalangeal joint (MTPJ) tenderness, particularly on the dorsal surface
- Unilateral versus bilateral involvement

Move

- Limited first MTPJ dorsiflexion
- May be associated with crepitus (see below)

Finish your examination here

Completion

Say that you would like to:

- Watch the patient walk
- Examine his shoes
- Ask him questions to assess the effect of the condition on his life

QUESTIONS

(a) What is hallux rigidus?

- Painful loss of motion (particularly dorsiflexion) of the first MTPJ secondary to degenerative joint disease
- May be due to bony degeneration, which can be either primary, as in osteoarthritis, or secondary to degenerative conditions, such as gout
- May be due to capsular damage and contraction

(b) What are the radiological changes associated with hallux rigidus?

- Initially normal
- Degenerative osteoarthritic changes seen later, particularly joint space narrowing and marginal osteophytes (especially dorsally and laterally)

(c) How would you treat this gentleman's condition?

Non-surgical:

- Appropriate footwear, e.g. stiff-soled shoes to limit dorsiflexion of the first MTPJ or rocker-bottom soles
- During acute exacerbations – use of nonsteroidal anti-inflammatories (NSAIDs) or intra-articular steroid injections for temporary relief – this is technically difficult if the spaces between the joints has narrowed

Surgical:

- Early disease (good range of movement and little loss of joint space) – cheilectomy (excision of dorsal segment of metatarsal head)
- Advanced disease – consider silastic interposition arthroplasty or arthrodesis

ADVANCED QUESTIONS

(a) What other diagnosis should you be aware of when managing a patient with hallux rigidus?

- Diffuse joint osteoarthritis – characterized by tenderness of the sesamoid bones and more crepitus than in hallux rigidus

(b) What is the optimal position for fusion of the MTPJ during arthrodesis?

The position of fusion should be tailored to the individual, but generally:

- 10–15° of dorsiflexion (with respect to the floor)
- 15° of valgus
- Neutral rotation

FURTHER READING

Shereff M J, Baumhauer J F (1998) Hallux rigidus and osteoarthrosis of the first metatarsophalangeal joint. *J Bone Joint Surg Am* **80**(6): 898–908

Weinfeld S B, Schon L C (1998) Hallux metatarsophalangeal arthritis. *Clin Orthop* **349**: 9–19.

http://www.medicalmultimediagroup.com/pated/foot/rigidus/rigidus.html – guide for patients to hallux rigidus

http://www.soarmedical.com/medical-library/foot&ankle/rigidus – good diagrams on this website which explain the condition well

---

** **CASTS** | **CASE 97**

INSTRUCTION

Patients with casts can easily be recruited from clinics for the clinical examination. Be prepared to describe casts and to discuss their advantages and complications.

Description of the cast

- Plaster of Paris or newer cast material (see below)
- Complete or incomplete (the latter is also known as a slab, or backslab)
- Positioning of the cast, such as above or below the joint. Remember that ideally the joints above and below the fracture should be immobilized in order to prevent displacement of the fracture
- Special casts, such as patella tendon bearing (Sarmiento) casts which allow movement of the knee while controlling the rotation of tibial fractures
- Has functional cast bracing been used? These are casts with hinges attached to allow some movement of the joint in a controlled manner. They are most commonly used for fractures of the tibia or femur. Functional cast braces can be:
  – simple, such as for the elbow
  – complex, e.g. polyaxial at the knee

Complications

Tight casts:

- Due to tight casting, ridges in the cast due to poor application or limb swelling. This may lead to vascular compression and compartment syndrome. Warn patients of the symptoms of compartment syndrome (see Notes) – if there is any suspicion that the cast is too tight, remove it

Loosening of the cast leading to failure of fixation

Skin complications:

- On application – pressure sores can occur particularly over bony prominences and are best prevented by adequate padding

- On removal – abrasions and lacerations can occur, especially if an electric saw is used
- Foreign body – may fall into the cast necessitating replacement
- Allergic reactions (rare)

Advantages of newer cast materials

- Lighter
- Stronger
- More radiolucent
- Waterproof
- Resistant to wear and tear
- Different colours available (for children)
- Less untidy to apply (than Plaster of Paris)

Disadvantages of newer cast materials

- Expense
- Skin irritation (gloves should be worn by the applicant)
- Less deformation after setting, therefore increased risk of neurovascular compromise if the limb swells
- More difficult to apply
- Can be very difficult to remove in an emergency situation without a proper plaster saw

Plaster of Paris – points of note

- Use first described by Antonius Mathijsen, a Flemish military surgeon, in 1854 for war injuries
- The name originates from the Montmartre region of Paris where it was first mined
- Consists of open-weave cloth or muslin strip impregnated with dehydrated calcium sulphate
- On addition of water, an exothermic reaction occurs, calcium sulphate becomes hydrated and rapidly sets
- Cloth is made stiffer using dextrose or starch
- Hardening rates can be altered using accelerators or inhibitors

Newer cast materials – points of note

- Knitted material of cloth or glass fibre impregnated with a monomer or polymer of polyurethane with substituted isocyanate terminal groups
- On addition of water the compound polymerizes and releases carbon dioxide
- Highly reactive material which is packaged in resistant containers

NOTES

- Compartment syndrome is defined as elevated compartment pressures within a soft-tissue envelope (either due to decreased space or increased pressure)

- Remember all the **P**'s for symptoms and signs
  - **P**ain out of **P**roportion to injury
  - **P**ain on **P**assive flexion
  - **P**alpate tense compartment
  - **P**allor, **P**aralysis, **P**araesthesia and **P**ulselessness (these are all seen late in the condition)
- The diagnosis is made clinically and can be confirmed with compartment pressure monitoring – with the latter, urgent treatment is needed if the absolute compartment pressure is greater than 30 mmHg or if the compartment pressure is within 30 mmHg of the diastolic blood pressure
- The treatment is emergency fasciotomy to decompress the involved compartments

---

** SIMULATED REDUCTION OF FRACTURES   CASE 98

INSTRUCTION

You may be asked to demonstrate the reduction of a common fracture (e.g. fracture of the distal radius) on a patient model – your understanding of the principles of fracture reduction is being examined, e.g. 'This lady has presented to you in Accident and Emergency with a fracture of the right distal radius which you have confirmed on X-ray views. I would like you to demonstrate how you would reduce this fracture in A&E.' You may be shown an X-ray of the fracture at this point.

APPROACH

Introduce yourself to the patient and begin by describing the fracture on the X-ray (the site of the fracture, any associated displacement, deviation or shortening, involvement of the ulna, etc).

VITAL POINTS

Initiation

- Place yourself on the same side of the patient as the injury
- Explain the fracture to her and the need for reduction
- Explain that you will provide pain relief with a combination of inhaled nitrous oxide and local haematoma block with local anaesthetic (or your own preferred choice of analgesia)

Assistance

- Tell the examiner that you would use him as an assistant and position his hands proximal to the fracture site in order to provide counter-traction (usually just distal to the flexed elbow)

Traction

- Demonstrate the way that traction is performed, but do not pull with any force – *do not harm the patient*
- Explain that the first manoeuvre is linear traction by yourself from distal to the fracture site – traction serves to relax the musculature around the fracture site due to stretching

Reduction

- The manoeuvres performed essentially serve to reverse the direction in which the fragment displaced at the time of injury and will depend upon the fracture itself, e.g. with dorsal displacement of the fragment, an opposing volar force is needed to effect the reduction. Sometimes it is necessary (while applying longitudinal traction) to actually increase the angulatory deformity in order to disimpact the fracture, and to then angle it down in the opposite direction.

Hold

- The fracture is held post-reduction in this case by a below elbow dorsal backslab (*not* a complete cast as swelling may occur post-application)
- A broad arm sling provides additional comfort

X-rays

- Anteroposterior and lateral X-rays are taken in order to check the reduction

Follow-up

- A fracture clinic appointment is made in 2–3 days time in order to check the reduction and complete the cast once the swelling has reduced
- It is particularly important to X-ray the wrist at 7–10 days as this is the most common time-point for the fracture to redisplace
- Say that you would like to give the patient an information leaflet on the care and complications of casts
- Explain that the fracture would normally take 4–6 weeks to heal, after which she may need physiotherapy for any resulting stiffness

Conclusion

- Thank the patient and turn to face the examiner

** LUMBAR DISC HERNIATION   CASE 99

INSTRUCTION

'This lady is complaining of pain in her lower back radiating down to her right leg. Ask her a few questions, examine her and tell me what you think the problem is.'

APPROACH

The ideal patient for this case would be one with a known lumbar disc prolapse in whom there are focal neurological signs to be elicited. Be as gentle as possible when examining the patient's back in order to minimize the chances of hurting her.

VITAL POINTS

Important features to extract are:

- Age
- Occupation
- Features of the pain, especially site, radiation, any history of injury, and relieving and exacerbating factors
- Neurological symptoms (e.g. weakness, numbness and paraesthesia) and their distribution
- Sphincter disturbance – bladder and bowel symptoms (unlikely in patients used for examination purposes)
- Effect on patient's lifestyle, e.g. work, sleep
- Previous treatments, e.g. use of analgesia, physiotherapy, caudal epidurals, operative intervention
- Explore other causes of back pain, e.g. diseases of the pancreas, abdominal aortic aneurysm, loin pain from renal causes

EXAMINATION

It is essential to examine the patient in her underwear so that the whole back and lower limbs are exposed. Start with the patient standing facing away from you and examine her gait first, then her back and finally, examine her lower limbs after asking her to lie down on the examination couch.

Gait

Half-shut knife position – patient leans forward with a painful, partially flexed back.

Look

- Skin – scars, sinuses
- From the side – loss of normal lumbar lordosis
- Posture – the 'sciatic list' is an involuntary attempt by the patient to reduce nerve root irritation by leaning to one side in an effort to open up the neural foramen

Feel

- Muscle – erector spinae muscle spasm/tenderness

Move

- Forward flexion – ask the patient to touch her toes; normally her fingertips should be able to reach to within 5 cm of the floor (estimate distance from bony landmarks, e.g. ankle or knee)
- Extension – normally 30°
- Lateral flexion – ask the patient to slide hand down outside of leg; normally 30° to each side
- Rotation – ask the patient to sit down (to fix the pelvis) and fold her arms across her chest; normally 40° to each side

Lie the patient supine

Straight leg raising (SLR)

- Demonstrates lumbosacral nerve root irritation
- With the knee fully extended, gently flex the hip and record the angle at which there is onset of pain. This angle is normally 80° and Lasegue's sign is positive if pain is felt in the back, buttock and thigh at less than 60°
- A feeling of tightness in the hamstring is not significant
- Crossed SLR – if SLR on unaffected side produces pain on the affected side, this suggests L4/5 lumbar disc protrusion (this is the most specific sign for lumbar disc herniation)

Sciatic stretch test (SST)

- Having extended the hip as above, dorsiflexion of the foot should induce further pain
- Flexing the extended knee relieves the pain

Neurological examination of the lower limbs

- Tone
- Power – test in particular for movements affected by the involved nerve roots
- Reflexes – knee/ankle/plantars
- Sensation – looking for specific dermatomal loss (see Table 27 and Fig. 37)

Table 27

Prolapsed disc	Involved nerve root	Distribution of sensory symptoms	Distribution of motor signs	Involved reflexes
L4/L5	L5	Lateral aspect of the leg and dorsum of the foot	Weakness of big toe extension and ankle dorsiflexion	None
L5/S1	S1	Lateral aspect of the foot and heel	Weakness of ankle plantarflexion and foot eversion	Ankle jerk

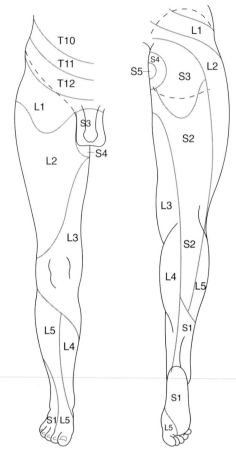

Fig. 37   Dermatomes of the lower limb.

Finish your examination here

Completion

Say that you would like to:

- Examine the patient prone – in particular, perform a femoral stretch test (FST) to exclude a L2/3/4 root lesion
- Examine the peripheral pulses – to exclude a vascular cause
- Examine the abdomen – to exclude intra-abdominal pathology that may cause back pain
- Perform a digital rectal examination – to check anal tone, perianal sensation and the anal reflex to exclude cauda equina compression (not likely to be encountered in the clinical examination!)

QUESTIONS

(a) What factors increase the risk of developing symptomatic disc degeneration and herniation?

Physiological:

- Increasing age
- Poor posture
- Poor overall aerobic fitness
- Poor strength of spinal extensor and abdominal muscles
- Decreased spinal mobility

Environmental:

- Smoking

Occupational:

- Heavy physical work
- Frequent bending, lifting, pushing, pulling and twisting
- Repetitive work postures
- Static work postures
- Vibration
- Psychological and psychosocial work factors

(b) How would you treat a lumbar disc herniation?

Non-surgical:

- Short period of bed rest (not more than 2 days) with appropriate analgesia (combination of muscle relaxant, nonsteroidal anti-inflammatories and opioids) for acute attacks
- Physiotherapy ('back school') aimed at muscle strengthening and stabilization, with emphasis usually on extension exercises, which strengthen back extensors and are less likely to increase intradiskal pressures

Epidural analgesia:

- Injection of a long-acting steroid with an epidural anaesthetic results in 60–85% short-term pain relief rate which falls to 30–40% at 6 months

Surgical – indicated with a herniated disc where there is a progressive neurological deficit and/or severe incapacitating pain (or failure of non-surgical treatment).

Options include:

- Chemonucleolysis of the disc with chymopapain – success rate ~70% but rarely used due to complications such as severe postoperative pain and spasms, and rarely, transverse myelitis and anaphylactic reactions
- Percutaneous diskectomy – decompresses the nerve root by removing disc material from the centre of the disc space; ~50% success rate
- Endoscopic diskectomy – success rates reported to be ~80% but technique still in evolution

- Open hemilaminotomy and diskectomy – gold standard with 85% success rate and performed with the use of loupe magnification or operating microscope

ADVANCED QUESTIONS

(a) What is the difference between sciatica and referred pain?

- The term sciatica should only be used to refer to nerve root pain in a specific *dermatomal* distribution
- Referred pain is pain caused by any lesion in a spinal motion segment which radiates distally in a *nondermatomal* pattern, e.g. to the buttocks, thighs, hips and occasionally the lower leg from the back. This pain is usually poorly localized, dull and less superficial than nerve root pain

(b) What is the pathology of disc herniation?

- Pre-existing degeneration contributes to disc herniation
- A disc consists of an outer annulus fibrosus and an inner nucleus pulposus
- Herniation is the end process of progressive rupture of the nucleus pulposus through the posterior annulus and herniation of this material into the spinal canal
- The initial pathology is asymptomatic disc fissuring and fragmentation
- This is followed by progressive annular disruption from the inner to the outer layers
- In some patients, this finally results in a complete annular rupture with herniation of disc material into the canal

FURTHER READING

Gibson J N, Grant I C, Waddell G (1999) The Cochrane review of surgery for lumbar disc prolapse and degenerative lumbar spondylosis. *Spine* **24**(17): 1820–32

http://www.worldortho.com/database/lectures/lecture3.html – an online lecture on low back pain

CASE 100   BRACHIAL PLEXUS LESIONS   *

INSTRUCTION

'This gentleman suffered an injury to his right upper limb 5 years ago in a road traffic accident. Ask him a few questions first, then examine him and tell me what you think.'

APPROACH

Ensure both upper limbs are fully exposed – ask him to take off his shirt if he has not already undressed. Note that the patient may have a mixed picture of upper and lower brachial plexus injuries (Fig. 38).

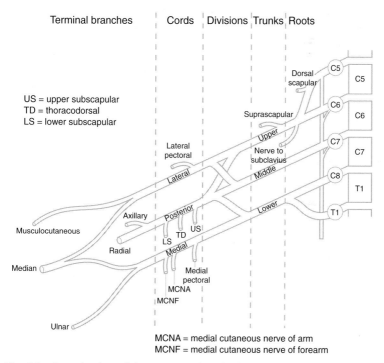

Terminal branches | Cords | Divisions   Trunks   Roots

US = upper subscapular
TD = thoracodorsal
LS = lower subscapular

Dorsal scapular
Suprascapular
Nerve to subclavius
Upper
Middle
Lower
C5, C6, C7, C8, T1

Lateral pectoral
Lateral
Posterior
Medial
Axillary
Musculocutaneous
Radial
Median
Ulnar
US, LS, TD
Medial pectoral
MCNA
MCNF

MCNA = medial cutaneous nerve of arm
MCNF = medial cutaneous nerve of forearm

Fig. 38   Organization of the nerves within the brachial plexus

VITAL POINTS

- Mechanism of injury:
  - if traction injury to the abducted arm, suspect lower brachial plexus lesion
  - if fall onto tip of shoulder, suspect upper brachial plexus lesion

- Clinical consequences – enquire about pain/sensory loss/paraesthesia/weakness
- Functional consequences – use of the limb for daily activities
- Previous treatments – ask about operative interventions, e.g. contracture release, nerve repair, tendon transfers
- Effect of the condition on the gentleman's quality of life and activities of daily living

Examination

You are essentially performing a neurological examination in order to distinguish between the various lesions.

Inspect

- Limb position
  - 'waiter's tip' position in Erb's palsy (Erb–Duchenne injury) C5 and C6 involvement – adducted shoulder, extended elbow, and forearm pronated and internally rotated
  - 'claw hand' in Klumpke's palsy (Dejerine–Klumpke injury) C8 and T1 involvement – paralysis of the small/intrinsic muscles of the hand
- Scars – traumatic/operative
- Muscle wasting/atrophy
- Fasciculations of involved muscles
- Inspect the face for evidence of ipsilateral Horner's syndrome (ptosis, anhydrosis, miosis and enopthalmos) (*see* Case 19)

Tone

- Flaccidity and hypotonia – lower motor neurone lesion

Power

- Compare power of muscle groups in affected limb to contralateral limb – note that in C5/6 lesions, there is decreased shoulder abduction and elbow flexion, while in C8/T1 lesions, there is decreased wrist flexion, and finger abduction and adduction

TOP TIP 1 – Nerve roots responsible for movements of the upper limb			
Shoulder abduction	C5	Wrist flexion	C7–8
Shoulder adduction	C5–7	Wrist extension	C7
Elbow flexion	C5–6	Finger flexion	C7–8
Elbow extension	C7	Finger extension	C7–8
		Finger abduction	T1

TOP TIP 2 – Medical Research Council grading of muscle power	
M0	No contraction
M1	Flicker or trace of contraction
M2	Active movement with gravity eliminated
M3	Active movement against gravity
M4	Active movement against gravity and resistance
M5	Normal power

Reflexes

• Hyporeflexia or absent reflexes in involved roots, e.g. biceps and supinator reflexes affected in C5/6 lesions

TOP TIP 3 – A way to remember limb reflexes (12345678!)	
S1/2	Ankle reflex
L3/4	Knee reflex
C5/6	Biceps and supinator reflexes
C7/8	Triceps reflex

Sensation

• Test light touch (cotton wool) and pain (orange stick) in all dermatomes compared with the unaffected side (Fig. 38):
  – in C5/6 lesions, the outer aspect of the arm (over the insertion of deltoid) is affected
  – in C8/T1 lesions, the ulnar side of the hand and forearm are affected

Completion

Say that you would like to:

• Determine whether the level of injury is more proximal than C5 – test trapezius (C3/4 root value) by asking the patient to shrug his shoulder against resistance
• Examine the neck to exclude compression from thoracic outlet syndrome, especially if there is no history of trauma (*see* Case 126)

QUESTIONS

(a) What are the branches of the brachial plexus? (Fig. 38)

• The brachial plexus is formed by the anterior rami of C5, 6, 7, 8 and T1 nerve roots (five roots)
• Three trunks – upper, middle and lower lying in the posterior triangle of the neck

- Six divisions – anterior and posterior division of each trunk at the level of the clavicle
- Three cords – lateral, medial and posterior formed as the 6 divisions enter the axilla (name of the cord denotes relationship to the axillary artery)
  - lateral cord – anterior divisions of upper and middle trunks
  - medial cord – anterior division of lower trunk
  - posterior cord – all 3 posterior divisions
- Nerve branches – remember the 3:1:0:3:5:5 rule (Table 28)

Table 28

3 from root	long thoracic nerve (C5,6,7)
	nerve to subclavius (C5)
	dorsal scapular nerve (C5,6)
1 from upper trunk	suprascapular nerve
0 from division	
3 from lateral cord	lateral pectoral nerve
	musculocutaneous nerve
	lateral contribution to median nerve
5 from medial cord	medial cutaneous nerve of arm
	medial cutaneous nerve of forearm
	medial pectoral nerve
	medial contribution to median nerve
	ulnar nerve
5 from posterior cord	upper subscapular nerve
	lower subscapular nerve
	thoracodorsal nerve
	axillary nerve
	radial nerve

(b) How would you differentiate between pre-ganglionic and post-ganglionic injuries?

Pre-ganglionic injuries have a worse prognosis as the nerve roots have been avulsed directly from the spinal cord and, as there is no proximal peripheral nerve tissue, surgical repair is impossible. The features of a pre-ganglionic injury are:

- Bruising in the posterior triangle of the neck
- Pain in an insensate hand
- Loss of sensation above the clavicle
- Ipsilateral Horner's syndrome (avulsion of C8/T1 nerve roots)
- Loss of muscle function of branches direct from the roots of the brachial plexus, e.g. long thoracic nerve (C5/6/7 – winging of the scapula) and phrenic nerve (C3/4/5 – elevated hemidiaphragm seen on chest X-ray)

ADVANCED QUESTIONS

(a) How would you assess the prognosis of a brachial plexus injury?

Three types of injury pattern have been described which provide a guide to prognosis:

- Root avulsion – direct avulsion of roots from spinal cord which is not amenable to surgical repair
- Rupture – of the plexus outside the vertebral column and although the injury is unlikely to heal spontaneously, surgery may be of some benefit
- Nerve damage without rupture – improvement likely to occur spontaneously

(b) What do you know of the staged management of brachial plexus injuries?

Staged management depends upon:

- Mechanism of injury, e.g. gunshot injuries – debride and treat as closed injury (see below)
- Whether the injury open or closed – if open, primary epineural repair and if closed, staged management
- Staged management is as follows:

  - stage I (3 months) – treat expectantly and assess clinically and electrophysiologically (electromyographic and nerve conduction studies)
  - stage II (3–6 months) – if clinical or electrophysiological improvement, continue to treat expectantly, if not, nerve exploration
  - stage III – nerve exploration and/or repair
  - stage IV – from time of exploration and repair to 1–2 years later (involves active hand therapy)
  - stage V (at 2 years) – final assessment of recovery made and adjunct procedures considered, such as tendon transfers, arthrodesis and amputation

---

Wilhelm Erb (1840–1921). German neurologist and Professor of Medicine at Leipzig and Heidelberg.
Guillame Benjamine Amand Duchenne (1806–1875). French neurologist.
Joseph Jules Dejerine (1849–1917). French neurologist and psychiatrist, and Professor of Neurology at the Salpetriere.
Johann Friedrich Horner (1831–1886). Professor of Opthalmology, Zurich, Switzerland.
Madame Dejerine-Klumpke née Auguste Klumpke (1859–1927). American-born neurologist married to Joseph Dejerine.

FURTHER READING

Terzis J K, Papakonstantinou K C (2000) The surgical treatment of brachial plexus injuries in adults. *Plast Reconstr Surg* **106**(5): 1097–122

Chuang D C (1999) Management of traumatic brachial plexus injuries in adults. *Hand Clin* **15**(4): 737–55

http://www.ninds.nih.gov/health_and_medical/disorders/brachial_doc.htm – information for sufferers of brachial plexus injuries

---

* **IVORY OSTEOMA**   **CASE 101**

INSTRUCTION

'Look at this gentleman's forehead and tell me the diagnosis.'

APPROACH

For the 'spot diagnosis' type question, simply introduce yourself to the patient as the examiner wants a quick answer to his question. Ivory osteomas are commonly found on the vault of the skull and frequently the forehead.

VITAL POINTS

Examine as for any lump (*see* Case 1)

Inspect

- Sessile, flat mounds

Palpate

- Smooth surface
- Bony hard in consistency
- Can move the superficial layers of the scalp across the top of the lump

---

TOP TIP – LAYERS OF THE SCALP
Remember the mnemonic that spells the word **SCALP**:
Skin
Connective tissue
Aponeurotic muscle
Loose areolar tissue
Periosteum

QUESTIONS

(a) What is an ivory osteoma?

Ivory osteomas are the most common benign tumours of the skull vault. They arise from cortical bone and radiologically may resemble sclerotic reaction produced by a meningioma (a CT scan may be needed to differentiate the two).

(b) How should they be managed?

They should not be resected unless they are symptomatic.

CASE 102   CHONDROMA   *

INSTRUCTION

'Examine this lump and tell me your diagnosis.'

APPROACH

Examine the relevant area – note that chondromas are usually found in the tubular bones of the hand or feet (e.g. phalanges).

VITAL POINTS

Examine as for lumps (*see* Case 1). Note that an enchondroma grows from the centre of the bone and an ecchondroma (periosteal chondroma) grows over the surface of the bone.

Inspect

- Visible solitary or multiple swellings
- May be fusiform (enchondroma) or sessile lumps (ecchondroma)

Palpate

- Smooth surface
- Hard consistency

QUESTIONS

(a) What is the differential diagnosis?

- Benign cysts (no calcification)
- Chondrosarcoma (older patients, especially in large bones)

(b) What is a chondroma?

- Benign cartilaginous tumours within or on the surface of long bones
- X-rays show well-defined lucent area in the medulla and characteristic specks of calcification

ADVANCED QUESTIONS

(a) What is the surgical treatment?

Surgical excision or curettage with bone grafting.

(b) What is Ollier's disease?

- Multiple chondromas (also known as dyschondroplasia) is a sporadic disorder with equal sex distribution where pathological fractures and growth arrest occur
- The rare combination of enchondromas with cutaneous haemangiomas is known as Mafucci's syndrome
- Patients with Ollier's disease have a 30% chance of developing malignant transformation to chondrosarcomas, and also have an increased risk of visceral malignancies.

> *A. Marfucci (1847–1903).* Professor of Pathology, Pisa, Italy.
> *L. Ollier (1830–1900).* French surgeon who was senior surgeon at the Hotel Dieu in Lyon in 1860.

FURTHER READING

Marco R A, Gitelis S, Brebach G T, Healey J H (2000) Cartilage tumors: evaluation and treatment. *J Am Acad Orthop Surg* **8**(5): 292–304

---

* CHARCOT'S JOINTS   CASE 103

INSTRUCTION

'Examine this gentleman's ankle.'

APPROACH

Compare both ankles, ideally by exposing the entire lower limbs, keeping the patient's underwear on.

VITAL POINTS

Look

- Look for swelling of the affected joint
- Colour of the overlying skin is usually normal

Feel

- Joint is not tender or warm (although it may have been in the early stages)
- Crepitus may be felt
- The normal contours of the joint are lost and the joint may be hypertrophic or atrophic
- The joint may be subluxed or dislocated

Move

- Instability of the joint may be demonstrated by abnormal movements and hypermobility

Finish your examination here

Completion

Say that you would like to:

- Perform a neurological examination of the affected limb, particularly looking for loss of sensation and joint position sense
- Dip the urine for sugar (to exclude diabetes mellitus)

QUESTIONS

(a) What is a Charcot's joint?

It is a progressive destructive joint arthropathy secondary to a disturbance of sensory innervation to a joint. The end result is a painless deformed joint resulting from repetitive minor trauma.

(b) What are the causes of a Charcot's joint?

Peripheral:

- Diabetic neuropathy
- Peripheral nerve injuries
- Leprosy

Central:

- Syringomyelia
- Cauda equina syndrome, e.g. secondary to myelomeningocoele
- Tabes dorsalis

> *Jean-Martin Charcot (1825–1893).* French neurologist and son of a Paris coachbuilder. Professor of Pathological Anatomy, Salpetriere Hospital in 1872. Subsequently the Professsor of Nervous Diseases in 1882, his pupils included Freud and Babinski.

FURTHER READING

Pinzur MS (2000) Charcot's foot. *Foot Ankle Clin* **5**(4): 897–912

http://www.diabetes.usyd.edu.au/foot/Chartec1.html – the radiological features of Charcot's arthropathy

* WINGING OF THE SCAPULA — CASE 104

INSTRUCTION

'Look at this gentleman's back and tell me your diagnosis.'

APPROACH

Expose fully to waist and ask the patient to turn around and face away from you.

VITAL POINTS

This case is essentially a spot diagnosis, and if asked to 'look at' the back do not touch the back.

Look

- Asymmetry of the shoulders (this may not be obvious until the patient pushes against a wall – see below)
- Any obvious scapular winging
- Bilateral involvement

Move

- Ask the patient to abduct his arm above the horizontal (there may be difficulty in performing this action)
- Ask him to stand up facing a wall and to push firmly with both hands against the wall (this makes winging more prominent and it is clinically easy to determine)

Finish your examination here

Completion

Say that you would like to examine the upper limb musculature to exclude muscular dystrophy.

QUESTIONS

(a) What is the most common cause of winging of the scapula?

Weakness of the serratus anterior muscle secondary to:

- Damage to the long thoracic nerve (anterior rami of C5, 6 and 7) which supplies serratus anterior, e.g. secondary to axillary surgery
- Upper brachial plexus injury
- Viral infections of C5, 6 and 7 nerve roots
- Certain types of muscular dystrophy, e.g. fascioscapulohumeral dystrophy (Dejerine–Landouzy syndrome)

ADVANCED QUESTIONS

(a) What other causes are you aware of?

- Trapezius palsy secondary to injury to the spinal accessory nerve (at risk of iatrogenic injury in the posterior triangle of the neck)
- Postglenohumeral fusion
- Abduction contracture of the deltoid

(b) How would you treat this condition?

- Non-surgical – if disability minimal
- Surgical – tendon transfers

Sir Charles Bell (1774–1842) – Scottish surgeon, physiologist and painter
J. J. Dejerine (1849–1917) – French neurologist
L. T. J. Landouzy (1845–1917) – French physician

FURTHER READING

Fiddian N J, King R J (1984) The winged scapula. *Clin Orthop* **185**: 228–36.

* EXTERNAL FIXATORS   CASE 105

INSTRUCTION

You may be shown an external fixator on a patient and asked to comment. The following notes are a guide to external fixators.

PRINCIPLES

- Focus – this is the area of bone being supported, i.e. the fracture
- Segment – this is the area of bone into which the external fixator is inserted in order to control the focus

The external fixator device is made up of pins and frame (the former connect the frame to the bone).

CLASSIFICATION OF PINS

External fixators are inserted into bone by:

(a) Screw-threaded half pins

- Applied to one side of the bone
- Advantage is the low risk of neurovascular damage
- But there is a risk of loosening

(b) Transfixing pins

- Passes through the bone from one aspect of the limb to the other
- Provides better control of the fracture
- Disadvantages include possible damage to neurovascular structures as the pins pass through the bone, and risk of loosening
- Therefore transfixing pins are only used in very simple constructs such as joint fusions and temporary stabilization of severely traumatized limbs.

(c) Tensioned fine wires

- Also pass all the way through the limb
- This support is made of multiple small, thin wires placed into the bone at different orientations which are then tightened to support the bone
- Are less traumatic to the blood supply of the limb and tend not to loosen but are more expensive and complicated to apply

CLASSIFICATION OF FRAMES

- Uni-axial – half pin (frame is adjacent to one side of the limb only)
- Circular – Ilizarov frame (frame circles around the limb)

- Hybrid – supports one segment using rings and other segments using uni-axial constructs
- Pinless – metal clamps that tighten onto the bone and therefore avoid interfering when the medullary canal when later definitive internal fixation is being considered

INDICATIONS

- Multiple trauma – there is evidence that adult respiratory distress syndrome may complicate intramedullary nailing when there has also been a concurrent chest injury, therefore external fixators are an alternative
- Peri-articular fractures
- Intra-articular fractures
- Open fractures
- Pelvic fractures – to reduce life-threatening haemorrhage
- Bone transport (Ilizarov technique) – for encouraging fracture union and replacing lost bone

COMPLICATIONS

- Pin-track infections
- Chronic pain
- Pin loosening and breakage
- Neurovascular damage
- Joint stiffness

Professor Gabriel Abramovitch Ilizarov graduated from medical school in the Soviet Union in 1943, near the end of World War II. After graduation, he was assigned to practice in Kurgan, a small town in western Siberia. He was the only physician within hundreds of miles and had little in the way of supplies and medicine. Faced with numerous cases of bone deformities and trauma victims due to the war, Professor Ilizarov used the equipment at hand to treat his patients. Through trial and error, with handmade equipment, this self-taught orthopaedic surgeon created the Ilizarov technique of distraction osteogenesis. This refers to the formation of new bone between two bone surfaces that are pulled apart in a controlled and gradual manner.

FURTHER READING

http://wheeless.belgianorthoweb.be/o16/92.htm – online orthopaedic textbook section on external fixators with useful diagrams and photos to help you familiarize yourself with various constructs

* INTRAMEDULLARY NAILS   CASE 106

INSTRUCTION

You may be shown an intramedullary nail, particularly one that has been removed from a patient (the nail is likely to be lying next to a patient or may be shown as a prop in between cases). You should be able to recognize the fact that it is an intramedullary nail and know some basic principles.

MATERIAL

- Most nails are made from stainless steel, titanium, or titanium alloys (e.g. titanium–aluminium–vanadium)
- Titanium and its alloys are stronger, lighter, more resistant to infection and osseointegrate better than stainless steel

LOCKING

Screws inserted proximally and distally:
- Provide longitudinal and rotational stability
- May be static or dynamic – in the former, the screws are inserted through round holes thus forming a fixed construct, whereas in the latter, some element of movement at the fracture site is allowed by locking one end of the nail or placing one screw through an oblong hole.
- Dynamization – this is the process of removing one or more screws in order to allow collapse, which increases the loading of the fracture site and hastens union

CONTROVERSIES OF REAMING

- Enlarges medullary canal and therefore permits insertion of the stronger, wider nail – this may not be necessary with modern materials
- Weakness due to the loss of endosteal bone
- Disturbance of medullary blood supply may cause cortical necrosis
- Time-consuming
- May cause embolism of debris into medullary veins – this is implicated in the aetiology of adult respiratory distress syndrome in severe trauma

FURTHER READING

http://www.medmedia.com/oa2/56.htm – general information on intramedullary nailing from an online orthopaedic textbook

CASE 107 — PAGET'S DISEASE OF BONE *

INSTRUCTION

'Have a look at this gentleman's legs.'

APPROACH

Expose the patient's legs but preserve his dignity by keeping his underwear on.

VITAL POINTS

Look

- Anterior bowing of the tibia (also known as sabre tibia)
- There may be lateral bowing of the femur

Feel

- The affected bone for warmth

Finish your examination here

Completion

Say that you would like to:

- Examine for the typical appearance of the skull – enlarged due to increased skull diameter (note that more than 55 cm is abnormal)
- Ask the patient if he has any hearing difficulties (either a conduction defect due to involvement of the ossicles or neural due to compression of the eighth nerve)
- Ask about osteoarthritic involvement of joints (e.g. limitation of hip abduction and fixed flexion deformity of the knees)
- Inspect the neck for a raised jugular venous pressure (cardiac failure secondary to a hyperdynamic circulation)
- Inspect the spine for kyphosis (and auscultate over the vertebral bodies for bruits – secondary to hyperdynamic circulation)

QUESTIONS

(a) What is Paget's disease?

Paget's disease is a remodelling disease of isolated skeletal areas – there is increased bone turnover with increased numbers of osteoblasts and osteoclasts with bone enlargement, deformity and weakness.

(b) What are the biochemical features of Paget's disease?

- Normal serum calcium and phosphate (occasionally hypercalcaemia)
- Markedly raised serum alkaline phosphatase (due to increased osteoblastic activity)
- Increased urinary hydroxyproline secretion (due to increased bone resorption)

(c) What are the complications of Paget's disease?

- Bone – increased risk of fractures, sarcomatous change (affects 1% of patients who have the disease for more than 10 years)
- Neurological – cranial nerve palsies, cord compression due to basilar invagination, nerve root lesions due to vertebral damage, headache, fits
- Cardiac – high-output cardiac failure

(d) How would you treat Paget's disease?

- Symptomatic – simple analgesics, progressing to bisphosphonates (e.g. alendronate), which inhibit osteoclast-mediated bone resorption. Calcitonins, which act by reducing osteoclastic activity, are less effective than bisphosphonates
- Surgical, e.g. hip arthroplasty for symptomatic osteoarthritis

ADVANCED QUESTIONS

(a) What are the radiological features of Paget's disease?

The hallmarks on plain X-rays are localized bony enlargement and patchy cortical thickening with sclerosis, osteolysis and deformity. More specific features include:

- Skull – 'honeycomb' and 'cottonwool' appearance with underlying osteoporosis circumscripta
- Vertebrae – 'picture frame' appearance due to sclerotic margins
- Pelvis – 'brim-sign' due to thickening of the iliopectineal line, enlargement of the ischial and pubic bones
- Long bones – increased trabeculation (note that bone scans are more sensitive for assessing the extent of disease)

(b) What do you know about the aetiology of Paget's disease?

Several theories exist including:

- Genetic – exact mechanisms unclear; some studies point to a recently identified candidate gene on chromosome 18q
- Infectious – may be due to slow viral infection, e.g. measles syncitial virus, paramyxovirus

(c) What changes can be seen on fundoscopy in patients with Paget's disease?

- Optic atrophy
- Angioid streaks – known as Terry syndrome

Sir James Paget (1814–1899). English Surgeon, St Bartholomew's Hospital, London and Professor of Surgery, Royal College of Surgeons. Described Paget's disease of bone as *osteitis deformans.* Also described:

- Paget's disease of the nipple – intra-epidermal, intraductal cancer involving the areola and/or the nipple characterized by large cells with a clear cytoplasm
- Paget's disease of the skin – skin cancer involving the apocrine glands characterized by large cells with a clear cytoplasm
- Paget–Schroetter syndrome – idiopathic axillary venous thrombosis
- Paget's sign (on testing whether a lump is fluctuant) – rest two fingers of one hand on opposite sides of the lump and press the middle of the lump with the index finger of your other hand – if the fingers are moved apart, the lump is fluctuant and you have demonstrated Paget's sign (*see* Case 1)

T. L. Terry (1899–1946). US opthalmologist.

FURTHER READING

Noor M, Shoback D (2000) Paget's disease of bone: diagnosis and treatment update. *Curr Rheumatol Rep* **2**(1): 67–73

Siris E S (1999) Goals of treatment for Paget's disease of bone. *J Bone Miner Res* **14** (Suppl 2): 49–52

http://www.paget.org/index.asp?p=Information%2Fdisease%5Ffr%5Fbottom%2Easp%23patients – information for patients

CASE 108   ACHONDROPLASIA   *

INSTRUCTION

'Have a look at this gentleman and describe what you see.'

APPROACH

Introduce yourself, step back and talk systemically through the physical appearance of the patient. Remember not to lay a hand on the patient unless the examiner prompts you to.

VITAL POINTS

Height

- Reduced (dwarfism, but avoid use of this word in the exam)
- Normal trunk size
- Shortened extremities

Hands

- Short and broad
- Wedge-shaped gap between middle and ring fingers (trident hands)

Skull

- Macrocephaly
- Frontal bossing (prominent forehead)
- Saddle nose (depression of the root of the nose)
- Maxillary hypoplasia
- Mandibular prognathism (protrusion of the jaw)

Spine

- Thoracolumbar kyphosis
- Excessive lumbar lordosis

Knees

- Genu varum

Finish your examination here

Completion

Say that you would like to:

- Take a family history (see below)
- Assess the effect of the symptoms on the patient's quality of life

QUESTIONS

(a) What is achondroplasia?

- Commonest form of disproportionate short stature with proximal shortening of long bones
- Equally common in males and females
- Prevalence is between 0.5 and 1.5 in 10 000 live births.

(b) What treatment options are available for the problems associated with achondroplasia?

Non-surgical:

- Subcutaneous human growth hormone to increase height
  - prominent height gain for 1 year
  - average of 7.5 cm height gain over 5 years
  - no beneficial effect > 5 years
  - large variation in effect between individuals

Surgical:

- Limb lengthening using distraction devices
  - correct body proportion and axial deviation
  - improve appearance, body-image and self-esteem
- Region-specific surgery, e.g.:
  - spinal surgery – correction of thoracolumbar kyphosis, decompression for spinal stenosis
  - correction of genu varum (by fusion of the fibular epiphysis or osteotomy)

ADVANCED QUESTIONS

(a) Do you know of any conditions resembling achondroplasia?

- Hypochondroplasia – similar to mild achondroplasia
- Pseudochondroplasia – similar to achondroplasia but normal head and face

(b) What do you know about the genetics of achondroplasia?

- Autosomal dominant with complete penetrance
- Around 80% of cases represent new mutations
- Mutations in transmembrane domain of fibroblast growth factor receptor 3 (FGFR-3) mapped to chromosome 4p16.3
- Transition from guanine to adenine or guanine to cytosine at nucleotide 1138

FURTHER READING

Baitner A C, Maurer S G, Gruen M B, Di Cesare P E (2000) The genetic basis of the osteochondrodysplasias. *J Pediatr Orthop* **20**(5): 594–605

http://www2.shore.net/~dkennedy/dwarfism_hgfachon.html – information for patients from the Human Growth Foundation

CIRCULATION AND LYMPHATIC SYSTEMS

CASE 109   VARICOSE VEINS   ***

INSTRUCTION

'Examine this lady's varicose veins.'

APPROACH

Expose the patient up to the groin, maintaining her dignity by keeping her external genitalia covered.

VITAL POINTS

Inspect

- Look at the legs with the patient lying down. Examine specifically around the medial malleolus (the 'gaiter' area) for the **complications** of varicose veins:
  - venous eczema
  - lipodermatosclerosis
  - ulceration – active and healed (the latter causing a white patch called *atrophie blanche*)
  - peripheral oedema
- Look for scars indicating previous surgery
- Stand the patient up and while kneeling in front of the patient, look for varicosities along the course of the long saphenous vein (LSV) (Fig. 39)
- Ask the patient to turn around and repeat for the short saphenous vein (SSV).
- Decide whether the varicosities are long or short saphenous in origin, commenting that the distinction may be difficult below the knee

Palpate

- Ask the patient to turn to face you again and palpate the saphenofemoral junction (SFJ) located two fingerbreadths below and lateral to the pubic tubercle (*see* Case 42)
- Feel for the smooth swelling and palpable thrill of a sapheno varix. If present, the cough test may be positive (Cruveilhier's sign)
- The Trendelenburg test (see Top Tip) is performed with the patient first lying down. Elevate the leg and gently empty the veins. Palpate the SFJ and ask the patient to stand while maintaining pressure. If the veins do not refill then the SFJ is incompetent. Should the veins fill, then the SFJ may or may not be competent, but there are certainly distal incompetent perforators
- The tourniquet test is similar but uses a tourniquet to control the junction rather than the fingers. It has the advantage that perforators can be examined below the groin by emptying the leg again and placing the tourniquet in the mid-thigh region (the test becomes less reliable below the knee)
- Use a hand-held Doppler (if provided) to identify SFJ/popliteal fossa reflux by squeezing the muscle of the thigh or calf, listening proximally as blood flows up the leg (normal) and then for a second 'swoosh' in incompetent veins as blood refluxes down the leg

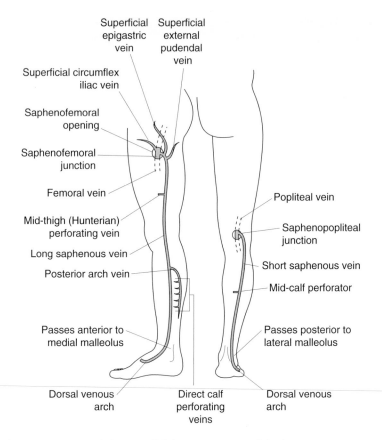

Fig. 39   Anatomy of the superficial venous system of the leg.

TOP TIP
The tourniquet test is easier to perform than the Trendelenburg test and we would recommend that this be performed in preference. Finish the examination after performing the first tourniquet test in the groin, simply telling the examiner that you could continue to examine lower down the leg for incompetent perforators.

Finish your examination here

Completion

Say that you would like to:

- Perform a tap test (Chevrier's tap sign)
- Auscultate the vein for bruits (indicating the presence of arteriovenous fistulae)

- Examine the abdomen for masses (including a digital rectal examination) to ascertain whether the varicose veins are primary or secondary

QUESTIONS

(a) What are the indications for pre-operative Duplex ultrasound scanning?

Some surgeons would advocate that all patients should undergo Duplex scanning of the leg veins before any surgery is undertaken. Others would consider indications to be:

- Previous history of deep vein thrombosis (DVT)
- Any ulceration (implies possible undiagnosed DVT)
- Recurrent varicose veins
- Difficulty in deciding whether the SSV or LSV is incompetent

(b) How would you treat varicose veins?

Non-surgical:

- Graduated elastic support stockings (Grade II compression)
- Encourage weight loss and regular exercise

Surgical:

- Injection sclerotherapy with 1% sodium tetradecyl sulphate (high recurrence rate) – indicated for:
  - postoperative recurrence of veins
  - below knee varicosities if the LSV and SSV are not involved
- Ligation of the incompetent SFJ or SPJ with stripping of the involved vein and stab avulsion of varicosities
- Ligation of incompetent perforating vessels (with site of incompetence preoperatively marked with Duplex)
- Subcutaneous endoscopic perforator surgery (SEPS)

(c) What would you tell this lady about the proposed surgery?

- Procedure usually performed as day case
- Need to wear tight-fitting stockings for 4 weeks postoperatively
- No driving for one week
- Does not alter the skin changes, including skin flares
- May not improve symptoms such as aching
- Risk of recurrent veins (20% at 5 years)

ADVANCED QUESTIONS

(a) What do you know about the pathophysiology of varicose veins?

Fibrous tissue invades the tunica intima and media of the vein and breaks up the smooth muscle, preventing the maintenance of adequate vascular tone. These changes are patchy and may not affect adjacent segments of vein.

(b) What syndromes are associated with varicose veins?

- Klippel–Trenaunay–Weber syndrome consists of a triad of varicose veins, port wine stains and bony and soft-tissue hypertrophy of the limbs. This may present with varicose veins in an unusual position, classically over the lateral aspect of the thigh. Peripheral oedema is often significant, as the deep venous system may be abnormal
- The Parkes–Weber syndrome is characterized by multiple arteriovenous fistulae, with limb hypertrophy. The AV fistulae may be so severe as to cause high-output cardiac failure

> *M. Klippel (1858–1942).* French psychiatrist and neurologist
> *P. Trenaunay* French neurologist
> *Professor F. Trendelenburg (1844–1924).* German surgeon, Leipzig
> *F. P. Weber (1863–1962).* British physician

FURTHER READING

Critchley G, Handa A, Maw A *et al.* (1997) Complications of varicose vein surgery. *Ann R Coll Surg Engl* **79**(2): 105–10.

Houghton A D, Panayiotopoulos Y, Taylor P R (1996) Practical management of primary varicose veins. *Br J Clin Pract* **50**(2): 103–5.

Pleass H C, Holdsworth J D (1996) Audit of introduction of hand-held Doppler and duplex ultrasound in the management of varicose veins. *Ann R Coll Surg Engl* **78**(6): 494–6.

http://www.utsurg.uth.tmc.edu/grand/vdisease/index.html – comprehensive guide (with illustrations) of varicose veins and associated surgery.

*** VENOUS ULCER   CASE 110

INSTRUCTION

'Examine this lady's ankle and tell me the diagnosis.'

APPROACH

The patient should be exposed from the groin to the toes, preserving her dignity.

VITAL POINTS

Look

Observe the following characteristic features of a venous ulcer

Site

- The venous ulcer is most commonly found over the lower third of the medial aspect of the leg, immediately above the medial malleolus ('gaiter area')

Shape

- The size varies enormously, and they can be extremely large

Edge and base

- The edge is sloping and pale purple/brown in colour; the base is usually covered with pink-coloured granulation tissue but there may also be some white fibrous tissue; they are usually rather shallow and often have a seropurulent discharge

Surrounding skin

- Look for signs of primary varicose veins
- The signs of chronic venous disease are usually present – induration, pigmentation, and brown discolouration of lipodermatosclerosis
- Oedema, spider veins and telangectasia may be present

Feel

- Feel the adjacent skin for temperature – it may be warmer than the rest of the leg (compared with the ischaemic ulcer where the surrounding skin will be cold)

Finish your examination here

Completion

- Ask the examiner to examine the limb properly for varicose veins (*see* Case 109)
- Mention that you would have to perform an ankle brachial pressure index measurement (*see* Case 111) as this must be > 0.8 before compression bandaging can be used

QUESTIONS

(a) What are the causes of venous ulcers?

Any cause of deep venous insufficiency can lead to ulceration:

- Valvular disease:
  – varicose veins
  – deep vein reflux (such as post-DVT)
  – communicating vein reflux (post-thrombotic or non-thrombotic) – controversial (unusual)
- Outflow tract obstruction:
  – often post-DVT
- Muscle pump failure:
  – primary – stroke, neuromuscular disease
  – secondary – due to stiff ankle

(b) How are venous ulcers treated?

Non-surgical:

- High success – 50–70% will heal at 3 months, 80–90% at 12 months
- The patient should be warned to avoid trauma to the affected area
- Four-layer compression bandaging comprising:
  - non-adherent dressing over ulcer plus wool bandage
  - crepe bandage
  - blue-line bandage
  - adhesive bandage to prevent the other layers from slipping
- Encourage rest and elevation of leg
- Once healed, Grade II compression stockings should be fitted and continued for life

Surgical:

- If the ulcer fails to heal, careful consideration should be given to excluding other causes (such as a malignant Marjolin ulcer) and the area may need to be biopsied (2% of chronic leg ulcers are malignant)
- Otherwise, a split skin graft should be considered with excision of the dead skin and the graft attached to healthy granulation tissue
- If ulceration is due to primary varicose veins, surgery to the superficial veins is required

---

Rene Marjolin (1812–1895). Surgeon in Paris who described the formation of a carcinoma in a chronic, non-healing ulcer.

FURTHER READING

London N J, Donnelly R (2000) ABC of arterial and venous disease. Ulcerated lower limb. *BMJ* **320**: 1589–91.

Fletcher A, Cullum N (1997) A systematic review of compression treatment for venous leg ulcers. *BMJ* **315**: 376–80.

CASE 111 — PERIPHERAL VASCULAR SYSTEM – EXAMINATION ***

INSTRUCTION

'Examine this gentleman's legs (from the point of view of the peripheral vascular system).'

APPROACH

Expose the patient's legs from the groin to the toes (Fig. 40), preserving his dignity by keeping his underwear on.

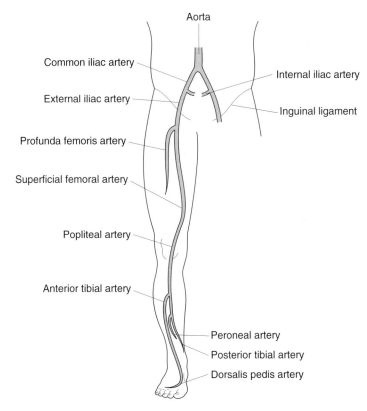

Fig. 40 Anatomy of the arteries in the leg.

VITAL POINTS

Look

Most of the pathology will be around the feet and toes. Begin by looking carefully at the feet. Observe the following features:

- Colour:
  – white/red
- Trophic changes:
  – loss of skin
  – loss of hair
  – gangrene (especially between and at the tips of the toes)
- Ulcers:
  – arterial (ischaemic) ulcers are found typically in the least well-perfused areas and over the pressure points, such as lateral aspect of foot and malleoli
  – the lesions are punched out (because there is no attempt at healing) and well described, may be very tender, and the surrounding skin is cold
  – they may vary considerably in size but are usually smaller than venous ulcers
  – there is no granulation tissue but may be a thin layer of slough at the base, otherwise the base is flat and pale
  – they may be very deep and penetrate surrounding tissue like bone
  – the commonest differential is with a neuropathic ulcer and if there is any doubt, the neurology should be examined
  – be sure to look between each of the toes on both feet
  – ask the patient for permission, then lift the foot up to observe the heel for ulcers (neuropathic ulcers are commonest here) and the sole of the foot for ulceration of the metatarsal heads
- Loss of digits, due to previous amputation

Feel

- First feel for skin temperature, keeping at the end of the bed next to the patient's feet – use the back of the hand, comparing one side with the other
- Examine the toes for capillary refill – use the thumb to push hard over the pulp of the big toe on both sides, normally the toe blanches but then returns to the normal colour within 2 seconds. This is not a very good test as refilling is mainly due to venous blood in the venules returning after the pressure is released
- Any longer than this is abnormal

Only after this has all been completed should you move on to examine the pulses.

Palpation of peripheral pulses

Many examiners like to begin with the radial pulse, to check for rate and rhythm.

Femorals:

- Move on from the radial to the femoral pulses, mentioning at the end that you would examine for an abdominal aortic aneurysm and the rest of the peripheral pulses

- The femoral pulse can roughly be identified by the level of the groin skin crease and should be palpated with the fingers parallel to the lie of the leg
- It is anatomically described at the mid-inguinal point, halfway between the anterior superior iliac spine and the pubic symphysis (*see* Case 42)
- Compare one side with the other

Popliteals:

- Move down to palpate the popliteal pulse, often quite difficult
- The pulse is demonstrated when the popliteal artery is compressed against the posterior aspect of the tibia
- Ask the patient to bend the knee slightly, and hold the knee between your hands. Use the pulps of your four fingers of both hands held alongside each other to feel the two heads of the gastrocnemius as they join (marking the lower borders of the popliteal fossa). The pulse lies between these two heads
- Again compare one side with the other

Foot pulses:

- The dorsalis pedis (DPA) and posterior tibial (PTA) pulses can be palpated bilaterally simultaneously
- Stand at the patient's feet and ask him to bring his big toe towards his head (thus demonstrating the tendon of extensor hallucis longus)
- The DPA is immediately lateral to this tendon
- Finally, swing your hands down to the medial malleolus on both sides and run your fingers posteriorly, demonstrating the pulse halfway between the medial malleolus and the heel

Listen

- Check for a bruit over the femoral artery and in the subsartorial canal

Finish your examination here

> TOP TIP
> This is a really good clinical case as most of the signs are elicited by looking at the foot alone. Much of the feel and move parts of the examination can be omitted in practice, but you should be able to describe the ankle brachial pressure index (as always never use the abbreviation 'ABPI'), and Buerger's test in detail – see below.

Completion

Tell the examiner you would:

- Examine the rest of the peripheral vascular system
- Examine the abdomen for an aneurysm
- Measure the ankle brachial pressure indices on each side

QUESTIONS

(a) How would you demonstrate this gentleman's ankle brachial pressure index?

- The pressure cuff is inflated over the upper arm and the systolic pressure measured at the brachial artery using a Doppler probe
- The cuff is then placed over the calf
- When the dorsalis pedis pulse has been located with the Doppler, the cuff is inflated until the pressure is high enough to occlude the artery and thus the Doppler sound disappears
- Slowly lower the cuff pressure until the Doppler sound restarts; this is the ankle pressure
- The index is the ankle pressure divided by the brachial pressure

(b) What is the significance of the ankle brachial pressure index?

- Normal index is 1
- As the perfusion of the leg begins to decrease in a patient with peripheral vascular disease, the ratio begins to fall
- Patients with intermittent claudication have a index of approximately 0.5–0.8
- Patients with rest pain have an index < 0.5
- An absolute pressure of less than 50 mmHg at the ankle is indicative of critical ischaemia

(c) How would you perform Buerger's test?

- Lifting the leg above the bed raises it above heart level if the patient is lying flat
- At some point the leg becomes white as the perfusion drops
- The angle between the horizontal and the leg when it becomes white is Buerger's angle
- Venous guttering can also be observed
- A normal leg can be raised to 90° and still remain perfused; if the angle is less than 20°, this indicates severe ischaemia
- Assisting the patient to drop their leg over the side of the bed causes the diseased leg to become purple-red in colour due to reactive hyperaemia – this is the second part of Buerger's test

> *Leo Buerger (1879–1943).* Austrian who lived in the USA all his life, became Professor of Urology in New York and subsequently Los Angeles. Also named Buerger's disease (thrombo-angiitis obliterans) (*see* Case 127).

CASE 112 — VASCULAR EFFECTS OF THE DIABETIC FOOT   ***

INSTRUCTION

'This gentleman has diabetes. Examine his foot and describe your findings.'

APPROACH

Expose the patient's legs from the groin to the toes, preserving his dignity.

VITAL POINTS

Look

Inspect the foot as for any vascular case (*see* Case 111). Diabetic peripheral vascular disease is usually below the knee in site. Note especially:

- Presence of bilateral disease
- Any previous surgical scars including excision of metatarsal heads or digits for ischaemic gangrene
- Charcot's joints are more common in diabetics with neuropathy (*see* Case 103)
- Signs of damage to the foot if the patient has a sensory neuropathy and cannot feel injuries such as hot bath-water or nails digging into the feet

Feel

- The pulses may be preserved until very late in the disease and may in fact feel quite prominent
- Take care when palpating the joints of the foot as they may be painful
- Test for sensation over the foot, and if any abnormality is detected, work proximally to find the level at which sensation returns to normal

Finish your examination here

Completion

- Ask the examiner whether he/she would like you to go on to examine the neurological system. Diabetic neuropathy is much commoner in Type 1 diabetics and can form a glove-and-stocking type sensory or mixed neuropathy. Isolated peripheral nerve lesions and autonomic neuropathy are also common in diabetes
- Don't forget to mention that you would examine the abdomen and the rest of the peripheral vascular system and if they do have Type 1 diabetes, fundoscopy is especially relevant, as is dipping the urine for proteinuria and testing for microalbuminuria as a marker of renal impairment

QUESTIONS

(a) Why are diabetics particularly prone to foot pathology?

Diabetic foot can be caused by:

- Neuropathy (microvascular)
- Peripheral vascular disease (macrovascular)
- Infection (both)

Diabetics are at 3–4 times the risk of the general population of having foot disease, and this is much higher if they smoke. Both Type 1 and Type 2 diabetics can have foot complications, although microvascular complications are commoner in Type 1. The natural history of their disease is also worse, because of a worse lipid profile, increased platelet aggregation and prothrombotic tendency. Their relative immunodeficiency leads to increased incidence of infection with *S. aureus* and *E. coli*, and slows healing.

(b) It is known that the pulses are preserved in the diabetic – why is this?

Calcification of the walls of the vessels preserves the pulses until late in the natural history of disease, and prevents the sphygmomanometer from compressing the vessels. This tends to lead to an abnormally (and reassuringly) high ankle brachial pressure index measurement. A similar effect is seen in peripheral vascular disease caused by chronic renal failure.

ADVANCED QUESTIONS

(a) What differences in management are there in diabetics?

The abnormal ankle brachial pressure index, plus the fact that patients often have occlusions at multiple levels, means that earlier recourse to intra-arterial digital subtraction angiography is indicated. Any infections should be treated aggressively with bed rest and intravenous antibiotics, together with meticulous foot care. Sepsis should be treated with surgical debridement. All diabetics should be seen regularly by the chiropodist with a view to preventing complications.

(b) Are there any problems with diabetics undergoing angiography?

They may have a degree of renal impairment which can be dramatically worsened following a dose of intra-arterial contrast. Patients should be kept well hydrated with intravenous fluids peri-procedure. If they are on metformin this has to be stopped prior to the procedure, as lactic acidosis has been reported.

FURTHER READING

Frykberg R G, Armstrong D G, Giurini J *et al.* (2000) Diabetic foot disorders: a clinical practice guideline. American College of Foot and Ankle Surgeons. *J Foot Ankle Surg* **39**(5 Suppl): S1–60.

Caputo G M, Cavanagh P R, Ulbrecht J S, Gibbons G W, Karchmer A W (1994) Assessment and management of foot disease in patients with diabetes. *N Engl J Med* **331**(13): 854–60.

CASE 113   AMPUTATIONS ★★★

INSTRUCTION

'Examine this gentleman's legs.'

APPROACH

- Expose the patient's legs from the groin to the toes, keeping his underwear or a gown in place
- The patient may be presented on a chair – if it is clear the examiner only wants you to look at the amputation, then the other leg should not be exposed

VITAL POINTS

Look

- Examine the amputation stump first
- Describe the anatomical level of the amputation, usually above-knee or below-knee
- If the patient has a partial foot amputation, then describe the level of amputation (Ray, transmetatarsal, Syme's)
- Comment on the stump – healthy stumps are cylindrical and the skin wound has healed completely
- Amputations are traditionally formed 12 cm above the knee or 14 cm below the knee
- Below-knee amputations can be performed in two ways:
  - long posterior flap of Burgess – posterior calf muscles are used to cover the transected bone, but the muscle should be debrided carefully so the flap is not too bulky to fit within the skin
  - skew flap of Kingsley Robinson – the suture line runs obliquely (anterior–posterior)
- In above-knee amputations, equal anterior and posterior semicircular flaps are formed – the vastus lateralis is sutured to the adductors, and the other quadriceps muscles to the hamstrings

Feel

The soft tissue under the skin should move freely over the bone beneath.

Move

- Ask the patient to actively flex and extend the knee joint immediately above the amputation to demonstrate the fixed flexion deformity that often follows a below-knee amputation if good physiotherapy has not prevented it
- Manipulate the joint passively if the patient cannot move it at all
- If the patient's prosthesis is available, ask to look at it, and then ask the patient to fit the appliance and walk with it in place

Finish your examination here

Completion

Tell the examiner that you would examine the rest of the limb and the other limb for signs of peripheral vascular disease.

QUESTIONS

(a) What are the indications for an amputation?

- Vascular:
  - peripheral vascular disease (80–90% of all cases)
  - thromboangiitis obliterans (*see* Case 127)
  - arteriovenous fistulae (*see* Case 131)
- Infection:
  - osteomyelitis
  - gas gangrene
  - necrotizing fasciitis
- Trauma:
  - burns
  - frostbite
- Malignancy

(b) What are the complications of amputations?

- Complications should be divided into specific to the amputation and general for any operation, and into immediate (within 24 hours), early (up to one month) and late (beyond one month)
- Mention at the beginning that these patients often have other medical problems, especially cardiovascular disease, putting them at particularly high risk
- Operative mortality is 20% and one-year survival is 50%

Specific early complications:

- Psychological and social implications
- Haematoma and wound infection, including gas gangrene (rare)
- Deep vein thrombosis and pulmonary embolism
- Phantom limb pain – due to the sensory cortex 'believing' the limb is still present
- Skin necrosis (caused by poor perfusion of the stump) requires refashioning, usually at a higher level

Specific late complications:

- Osteomyelitis – infection transmitted to the bone through the stump
- Stump ulceration – can be caused by pressure from the prosthesis
- Stump neuroma – swelling of the distal nerve as it tries to regrow following division; during the initial procedure the nerve should be cut back far enough to prevent a neuroma from forming
- Fixed flexion deformity of the knee, especially with long-term disease
- Difficulty in mobilizing
- Spurs and osteophytes in the underlying bone

> *James Syme (1799–1870).* Professor of Surgery, Edinburgh and University College Hospital, London, and father-in-law to Joseph Lister.

FURTHER READING

Dormandy J, Heeck L, Vig S (1999) Major amputations: clinical patterns and predictors. *Semin Vasc Surg* **12**(2): 154–61.

Robinson K P, Hoile R, Coddington T (1982) Skew flap myoplastic below-knee amputation: a preliminary report. *Br J Surg* **69**(9): 554–7.

http://www.medmedia.com/o13/44.htm – an online Orthopaedic textbook with further information on amputations and prostheses.

http://www.arch.gatech.edu/crt/Techknow/MedConditions/Amputation.htm – patient resource for information on life after amputation.

CASE 114   PERIPHERAL VASCULAR SYSTEM –   *
HISTORY**

INSTRUCTION

'This patient is describing some pain in the calf on walking. Ask him some questions to help you define the cause.'

APPROACH

Within a short case or OSCE, you may be asked to take a history from a patient, and vascular long cases are extremely common in the final MB examination.

VITAL POINTS

The history should be structured to answer three basic questions, summarized in Table 29.

Table 29

Vascular symptoms	Risk factors for arterial disease	Fitness for surgery
Intermittent claudication	Smoking	Previous medical history
Rest pain	Diabetes	Anaesthetic history
Critical ischaemia	Hypertension	Drug history and
	Cholesterol	allergies
	Previous history	Social history (related
	(especially heart	to postoperative
	disease or stroke)	rehabilitation)
	Family history	
	(Renal failure)	
	(Hypothyroidism)	
	(Gout)	

Introduction

- Ask the patient's age
- Ask their occupation

Pain of intermittent claudication

Site:

- Stenosis of the lower aorta and common iliac artery cause buttock claudication (and may be associated with impotence)
- External iliac artery stenosis causes thigh claudication
- Superficial femoral artery stenosis leads to calf claudication

Intensity:

- The pain is always felt in the muscles as it is due to increased oxygen demand from actively contracting muscle
- When the demand is not met due to ischaemia in the afferent arterioles, anaerobic metabolism takes over and lactic acidosis occurs
- The pain is due to anoxia, acidosis and the build-up of metabolites

Precipitating and relieving factors:

- The pain comes on during exercise and typically after a fixed distance
- It comes on more rapidly after walking up a hill rather than on the flat
- The pain is relieved after a few minutes of resting

Rest pain

Site:

- Rest pain is described in the least well perfused areas of the leg, over the toes and forefoot

Intensity:

- The pain is very severe, aching in nature and typically wakes the patient from sleep

Precipitating and relieving factors:

- The pain comes on at night when the patient is lying flat in bed
- It is relieved by getting up and walking on a cold floor and sometimes the patients describe that they have to sleep sitting up to prevent the pain from coming on
- Characteristically, the pain is also relieved by hanging the foot over the edge of the bed

Critical ischaemia

It is important to distinguish immediately whether there is any feature in the history which suggests more severe (limb-threatening) disease. Ask specifically about the presence of ulcers or gangrene ('trophic changes').

Critical limb ischaemia is defined by the European working group as:
(i)   Presence of arterial ulcers or gangrene, OR
(ii) Rest pain that lasts for two weeks or more and is only relieved by opiate analgesia, AND
(iii) An absolute ankle pressure (*see* Case 111) of less than 50 mmHg

Function

As for the orthopaedic history:

- Impact on patient's life, e.g. work, sleep
- Going to the shops
- Walking aids
- Limp

QUESTIONS

(a) What is the differential diagnosis of intermittent claudication?

The causes of pain in the leg can be divided into:

- Musculoskeletal – pathologies of the knee, ankle or hip (such as osteoarthritis)
- Neurological – spinal stenosis (leading to spinal claudication)
- Vascular – intermittent claudication, deep vein thrombosis

(b) Why do patients with rest pain typically get more severe pain at night?

The pain is caused by a reduced blood supply to the distal aspects of the limb. The pain gets worse at night because the perfusion of the limb is further reduced when the patient is lying down. This is due to:

- Decreased cardiac output at night
- Reduced effect of gravity, which normally acts to increase relative blood supply to the legs
- Relative dilatation of the skin vessels due to the warmth of the bedclothes

*** **ABDOMINAL AORTIC ANEURYSM** **CASE 115**

INSTRUCTION

'Examine this gentleman's abdomen.'

APPROACH

Expose the patient as for the abdominal examination (*see* Case 43).

VITAL POINTS

Inspect

- A midline pulsating mass may be visible, especially in deep inspiration – this is easier to identify in thin patients
- Note the presence of any abdominal scars

Palpate

- Hand examination is likely to be normal, and the examiner will probably move you on immediately to palpation of the abdomen
- Gentle palpation of the nine abdominal areas may be normal
- A pulsatile mass may be identified on deeper palpation in the epigastric region
- The mass should be measured by bringing the lateral sides of the index fingers of both hands together to identify the borders of the aneurysm and estimating the distance between your fingers (in cm)
- An expansile mass moves your fingers laterally with each pulse; aneurysms are expansile as well as pulsatile (a transmitted pulsation is not expansile – *see* Case 1)
- Take care not to palpate too firmly
- Palpate over the course of the common iliac arteries
- Continue the examination by palpating the femoral arteries in the groin and the popliteal arteries (which may also be aneurysmal in nature)

Auscultate

- For aortic and iliac bruits

Finish your examination here

> TOP TIP
> A common error is to try to palpate for an abdominal aortic aneurysm (AAA) too low. The abdominal aorta bifurcates at the level of L4, immediately below the umbilicus. Begin by palpating in the epigastric region to avoid missing the pulsation.

Completion

Say that you would like to examine the heart, carotid vessels and legs for concurrent cardiac, carotid or peripheral vascular disease.

QUESTIONS

(a) In which patients are abdominal aortic aneurysms most common?

Aneurysms are most common in:

- Men
- Aged > 60 years
- Smokers
- Hypertensive patients
- Often strong family history

(b) Which patients should have their aneurysms repaired?

- The reason for repairing abdominal aortic aneurysms is to avoid complications
- The following aneurysms should be repaired:
  - symptomatic aneurysms
    (back pain, tenderness over the aneurysm on palpation, distal embolic events, ruptured/leaked aneurysms)
  - asymptomatic aneurysms (≥ 5.5 cm diameter; increase of diameter of ≥ 1 cm per year, suggesting rapidly expanding aneurysm)
- The UK Small Aneurysm Trial suggests that if the aneurysm is between 4.0 and 5.5 cm in diameter, open surgical repair is not recommended, and for those greater than 5.5 cm in diameter, the patient will benefit from surgery
- The risk of rupture of a > 5.5 cm aneurysm is 10% per year, increasing with the size of the aneurysm

(c) What is the operative mortality of AAA repair?

- The elective mortality from open AAA repair is 5%, but this figure may be lower in specialist centres
- If the patient suffers a ruptured aneurysm and reaches the hospital, their operative mortality rises to 50%, but only 50% of patients reach hospital alive
- Mortality is usually from haemorrhage, subsequent myocardial infarction or renal failure

ADVANCED QUESTIONS

(a) Are there any other options other than open AAA repair?

- Endovascular repair, using grafts placed into the abdominal aorta from the femoral artery by a vascular surgeon and a radiologist, has been used over the last few years but the technique has not been perfected
- Although the operative mortality is lower, there is no long-term data to suggest that outcome is better from this procedure and there is a significant failure rate (approximately 25%), and medium-term complications like endoleaks are of increasing concern

- Laparoscopic repair of abdominal aneurysms is the subject of current clinical trials.

(b) Should we be screening for AAA?

- A screening programme in the UK has never been agreed, and opinions differ as to the value of screening on a population basis
- Lindholt *et al.* (2001) have shown that a single ultrasound screen of men at the age of 65 decreased the risk of death from rupture by 42%

(c) Do you know of any infectious agents associated with AAA?

- *Chlamydia pneumoniae* has been shown to be associated with AAA (and also atherosclerosis and myocardial infarction)
- A high proportion of males with AAA have signs of infection with *Chlamydia pneumoniae*
- The progression of their AAA has been positively correlated with the presence of indicators of *Chlamydia pneumoniae* infection.

FURTHER READING

Lindholt J S, Ashton H A, Scott R A (2001) Indicators of infection with Chlamydia pneumoniae are associated with expansion of abdominal aortic aneurysms. *J Vasc Surg* **34**(2): 212–5.

Scott R A, Vardulaki K A, Walker N M, Day N E, Duffy S W, Ashton H A (2001) The long-term benefits of a single scan for abdominal aortic aneurysm (AAA) at age 65. *Eur J Vasc Endovasc Surg* **21**(6): 535–40.

The UK Small Aneurysm Trial Participants (1998) Mortality results for randomised controlled trial of early elective surgery or ultrasonographic surveillance for small abdominal aortic aneurysms. *Lancet* **352**(9141): 1649–55.

http://www.medicinenet.com/Script/Main/Art.asp?li=MNI&ArticleKey=1951 – information for patients.

http://www.med.stanford.edu/school/surgery/html/vascular/case/case01.html – an online pictorial case showing the procedure for endovascular stenting.

Note

The actor George C. Scott died from a ruptured abdominal aortic aneurysm in September 1999, as did Sir John Hunter (*see* Case 117).

CASE 116   CAROTID ARTERY DISEASE   ★★★

INSTRUCTION

'Listen to this gentleman's neck.'

APPROACH

Expose the patient's neck as for the neck exam (*see* Case 6).

VITAL POINTS

This is a directed instruction and you should proceed immediately to auscultation

AUSCULTATE

- Notice the bruit over one or both carotid arteries
- The bruit is best heard over the course of the common carotid artery, which runs behind and medial to the sternocleidomastoid in the anterior triangle of the neck
- The bruit is best heard in expiration
- Tell the examiner that you would listen over the precordium to ensure this is not a transmitted aortic stenosis murmur (heard as an ejection systolic murmur in the aortic area – second intercostal space immediately to the right to the sternum).

Finish your examination here

TOP TIP
- The subject of carotid bruits and cerebrovascular events may also be brought up by asking you to question the patient with regards to his bruit
- In this case, you should ask about previous transient ischaemic attacks or stroke, asking about temporary or resolving neurological symptoms such as weakness or paraesthesia
- Also ask about amaurosis fugax, the visual sensation of a curtain being drawn down slowly in front of one eye
- Neurological symptoms occur on the contralateral side but amaurosis fugax is ipsilateral to the side of the carotid stenosis

---

Completion

You would perform a neurological examination to look for signs of a previous cerebrovascular event, and would also check for signs of atherosclerosis elsewhere (heart, abdominal aorta and peripheral vascular system).

QUESTIONS

(a) How would you investigate a patient who was referred with a carotid bruit?

The patient should have a full workup for atherosclerosis:

General investigations:

- Urinalysis for proteinuria, marker of atherosclerotic renal disease
- Blood tests
  - haematology: full blood count for anaemia, which might precipitate symptoms
  - biochemistry: renal function for possible undetected renal disease
  - glucose: exclude diabetes
  - cholesterol: to identify hypercholesterolaemia
- Electrocardiogram: To look for evidence of atrial fibrillation, cardiac disease, previous infarction, ischaemia or left ventricular dysfunction

Special investigations:

- A carotid duplex scan, looking for atherosclerotic plaques
- The report would detail the size and location of plaques, the diameter of the patent lumen remaining, and may also provide some information on the plaque friability or likelihood of embolization
- Carotid angiography to identify the anatomy of the carotid arteries in more detail is also a possibility, but this procedure in itself carries a 2% risk of stroke
- An echocardiogram would also be an option, especially if the patient had a precordial bruit
- A CT or MRI scan of the brain may be performed, demonstrating lacunar infarcts

(b) What is the consequence of carotid stenosis?

- Stroke is the third leading cause of death in the west and 85% of strokes are thromboembolic, caused by atherosclerosis at the carotid bifurcation or proximal (2–3 cm) internal carotid artery
- Atherosclerosis can also affect the intracranial circulation, particularly the circle of Willis and the vertebrobasilar system
- Transient ischaemic attacks (neurological symptoms resolving completely within 24 hours) and amaurosis fugax are usually caused by repeated microemboli from the plaque, consisting of clusters of platelets and cholesterol
- The same symptoms can be caused by microemboli from the heart and aortic arch

ADVANCED QUESTIONS

(a) Which patients might be considered for carotid endarterectomy (Fig. 41)?

- Symptomatic carotid stenosis of ≥ 70%
- Both the North American (NASCET, North American Symptomatic Carotid Endarterectomy Trial) and European (ECST, European Carotid Surgery Trial) trials set up to look at evidence-based reasons for carotid endarterectomy

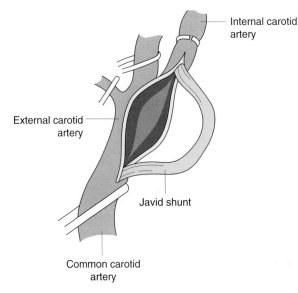

Fig. 41   Carotid endarterectomy.

demonstrated the value of surgery in patient with symptomatic stenosis of 70% or more

- These trials demonstrated that for patients with severe stenosis (over 70%) surgery reduced the relative risk of disabling stroke or death by 48%
- The benefit in asymptomatic patients has not yet been proven

(b) What would you warn the patient of in consenting them for an endarterectomy?

- The advantages of having surgery are a 6-fold reduction in the rate of stroke at three years
- The operative risk of stroke is 2% and operative mortality 1–2%
- Specific risks of haematoma, hypoglossal nerve injury, and numbness of the ipsilateral earlobe should also be mentioned

---

Thomas Willis (1621–1675). English physician and anatomist who described the sweet taste of diabetic urine, myasthenia gravis, general paralysis of the insane, whooping cough and identified the intercostal, spinal and spinal accessory nerves. He gave names to 'reflex' and 'neurology' and was buried in Westminster Abbey.

FURTHER READING

Cina C S, Clase C M, Haynes R B (2000) Carotid endarterectomy for symptomatic carotid stenosis. *Cochrane Database Syst Rev* 2: CD001081.

Randomised trial of endarterectomy for recently symptomatic carotid stenosis: final results of the MRC European Carotid Surgery Trial (ECST). *Lancet* **351**(9113): 1379–87.

North American Symptomatic Carotid Endarterectomy Trial (NASCET) investigators (1991) National Institute of Neurological Disorders and Stroke Stroke and Trauma Division. Clinical alert: benefit of carotid endarterectomy for patients with high-grade stenosis of the internal carotid artery. *N Engl J Med* **22**(6): 816–7.

** **POPLITEAL ANEURYSM** CASE 117

INSTRUCTION

'Examine the pulses in this gentleman's legs.'

APPROACH

Expose the patient's legs from the groin to the toes, preserving his dignity. If asked to examine the pulses, rather than the limb, be sure to begin by palpating the femoral pulse – you have not been asked to examine the feet for signs of peripheral vascular disease.

VITAL POINTS

Palpate the leg pulses

- Begin with the femoral pulses, comparing one side with another (*see* Case 111)
- Comment on whether the pulses are present or absent and whether the character of the pulse is normal
- Move down to the popliteal pulses
- Note the expansile pulsation behind the knee
- The aneurysmal pulse is relatively easy to find and the artery does not need to be compressed against the tibia
- Slide the fingers of your two hands apart and comment on the diameter of the vessel. A popliteal aneurysm is 2 cm or greater in diameter, although 1.8 cm is quoted as the cut-off for surgery
- The pulsating mass does not alter with change in position of the knee
- The ankle and foot pulses may not be palpable if the aneurysm is thrombosed
- 50% are bilateral – don't forget to examine the other knee

Finish your examination here

Completion

- Tell the examiner that you would examine the rest of the limb and the other limb for signs of peripheral vascular disease
- Ask to examine the abdomen as 50% will also have an abdominal aortic aneurysm

QUESTIONS

(a) How might a patient with a popliteal aneurysm present?

- Popliteal aneurysms represent 70% of all non-aortic aneurysms
- The patient may have presented with a lump behind the knee if the aneurysm has grown to such a size that it has expanded beyond the popliteal fossa
- 50% present with distal limb ischaemia caused by thrombosis or embolism
- Patients may present with an acutely ischaemic leg
- Less than 10% rupture

(b) Under what circumstances would they be treated?

Surgery is indicated for:

- Symptomatic aneurysms
- Those containing thrombus
- Those greater than 1.8 cm

The aneurysm is surgically repaired by either an excision bypass, where the popliteal artery is ligated above and below the diseased segment and a graft interposed, or a simple resection and anastamosis without the use of a graft (Hunter's ligation).

Acute ischaemia caused by thrombus can be treated with thrombolysis.

Sir John Hunter (1728–1793). Scottish Surgeon and Anatomist. Also described Hunter's canal (subsartorial adductor canal) and Hunterian chancre (syphilitic chancre). Interestingly, he died of a ruptured abdominal aortic aneurysm and was buried in Westminister Abbey.

FURTHER READING

Thompson M M, Bell P R (2000) ABC of arterial and venous disease. Arterial aneurysms. *BMJ* **320**(7243): 1193–6.

INSTRUCTION

'Examine this gentleman's feet.'

APPROACH

Again, ideally expose the whole of the legs from the groin, maintaining the patient's dignity, but if the patient is in an environment where other patients are present, this would be inappropriate and you should just comment on the feet.

VITAL POINTS

Begin examining the legs as for the peripheral vascular system examination (*see* Case 111).

Look

Observe the following characteristic features of an ischaemic ulcer.

Site:

- Characteristically over the tips of the toes and over the pressure areas

Shape:

- The size of the ulcer varies from a few millimetres on the tip of the toes to several centimetres over the lower leg

Edge and base:

- The edge is punched out, clean cut because there has been no partial healing of the wound
- The base may contain slough and may be infected but there is no healthy red granulation tissue as the blood supply is too poor
- The ulcer may be very deep and penetrate down to bone and the underlying joints – the bone may be exposed at the base

Surrounding skin:

- The skin around the ulcer is a grey/blue colour

Feel

- Palpate for temperature using the back of the hands – note the surrounding skin is cold compared with the proximal limb and the contralateral foot
- Check the peripheral pulses, noting the most distal pulse that is still palpable
- Check the pulses of the other leg

Finish your examination here

> TOP TIP
> Almost all of the examination is 'Look' and you should spend as much time as possible commenting on the features without progressing to 'Feel' as this will score marks very quickly.

QUESTIONS

(a) What are the causes of ischaemic ulcers?

These can be divided into large and small vessel arterial disease:

- Large vessel
  - atherosclerosis
  - thromboangiitis obliterans (*see* Case 127)
- Small vessel
  - diabetes mellitus
  - polyarteritis nodosa
  - rheumatoid arthritis

(b) What kinds of analgesia would be appropriate for this patient?

- Ischaemic ulcers can be extremely painful and even removing the bandages from around the ulcer can cause pain that lasts for several hours
- Consider the analgesic ladder (Table 30), remembering that combinations of drugs administered regularly in a variety of different formulations (oral, intramuscular etc) can be more effective

Table 30   The analgesic ladder

Stage	Analgesia
I	Simple, oral agents such as paracetomol or non-steroidal anti-inflammatory drugs (NSAIDs) like ibuprofen – taking great care in the elderly and patients with renal impairment – selective cyclooxygenase 2 (COX-2) inhibitors such as rofecoxib are also available which reduce the incidence of gastrointestinal bleeding
II	Stronger oral agents, such as a mixture of orally acting opioids like codeine and paracetamol
	Stronger NSAIDs such as diclofenac
III	Intramuscular, stronger oral or intravenous opioids such as morphine, diamorphine

(c) What other non-surgical treatments are available?

Risk-factor modification:

- Stopping smoking
- Good diabetic and hypertensive control
- Optimized serum lipid levels

Symptom modification:

- Avoidance of drugs which might worsen symptoms, such as beta blockers
- Commencement of low-dose aspirin (75 mg/day), which reduces the incidence of cardiac and cerebrovascular events in high-risk patients
- Intravenous prostaglandins act by inhibiting platelet aggregation, stabilizing leucocytes and endothelial cells, and are vasodilators. They can have some effect in healing ulcers, relieving rest pain and reducing the risk of amputation
- Lumbar sympathectomy reduces sympathetic-mediated vasoconstriction and improves perfusion by allowing for unopposed vasodilatation of the skin vessels. This is often unsuccessful in diabetics who may have autonomic neuropathy causing 'autosympathectomy'

Table 31   Comparison of different types of leg ulcer

	Venous	Ischaemic	Neuropathic
Site	Gaiter region over medial malleolus of ankle	Tips of toes and pressure areas	Heel, underneath metatarsal heads (pressure bearing areas)
Shape	Variable, usually irregular	Regular outline	Regular outline, follows skin contour
Size	Can be very large	Varying size, few mm to several cm	Several cm
Edge	Usually sloping pale purple/brown	Punched out, clean	Clean
Base	Pink granulation tissue or white fibrous tissue characteristic	Bone may be exposed, no granulation tissue	Often exposing bone
Surrounding skin	Chronic venous signs, e.g. lipodermatosclerosis	Grey/blue	Normal
Skin temperature	May be warmer	Cold	Normal
Pulses	Present	Absent	Present

FURTHER READING

Sarkar P K, Ballantyne S (2000) Management of leg ulcers. *Postgrad Med J* **76**(901): 674–82.

London N J, Donnelly R (2000). ABC of arterial and venous disease. Ulcerated lower limb. BMJ **320**(7249): 1589–91.

Note

About 400 years BC, Hippocrates wrote, 'In case of an ulcer, it is not expedient to stand, especially if the ulcer be situated on the leg'. Hippocrates himself had a leg ulcer.

CASE 119   POST-PHLEBITIC LIMB   **

INSTRUCTION

'Examine this gentleman's legs.'

APPROACH

Expose the patient's legs, maintaining his dignity and keeping his underwear on. Ensure that you can see his feet, and position him lying comfortably on the couch.

VITAL POINTS

Look

Note the features of chronic venous insufficiency, comparing one side with the other:

- Swelling
- Dilated superficial veins (as blood cannot return to the inferior vena cava through the deep veins)
- Skin pigmentation, possibly restricted to the medial malleolus ('ankle flare')
- Venous eczema
- Lipodermatosclerosis
- Venous ulceration or evidence of previous ulceration

Feel

- Compare the temperature of both legs
- Check for pitting oedema (watching the patient's face at all times)

Finish your examination here

Completion

Say that you would like to:

- Test for deep venous occlusion – Perthe's test – place a high tourniquet around the top of the patient's thigh and ask them to walk. If the deep venous system is occluded, the leg will become swollen and blue with dilated superficial veins distal to the tourniquet

ADVANCED QUESTIONS

(a) What is venous gangrene?

Venous gangrene is a rare complication of deep vein thrombosis in the iliofemoral segment and presents in three phases:

1. Phlegmasia alba dolens (white leg)
2. Phlegmasia cerulea dolens (blue leg)
3. Gangrene – occurs as a consequence of acute ischaemia and may be restricted to the foot or spread up the leg

(b) What investigations are appropriate for deep venous disease?

- Duplex – shows areas of reflux and deep venous occlusion
- Venography:
  - ascending – identifies deep venous patency and perforator incompetence
  - descending – identifies areas of reflux
- Varicography – shows sites of communication
- Ambulatory venous pressures ('gold standard' investigation)

(c) What are the surgical options available for deep venous occlusion/reflux?

Reflux:

- Tahere transplantation – use a segment of axillary vein with valve and insert it into the deep venous system of the leg, wrapping it in a PTFE cuff
- Kistner's operation – valvuloplasty of damaged valves

Obstruction:

- Palma operation – use contralateral long saphenous vein (LSV) and anastamose to the femoral vein to bypass iliofemoral obstruction
- Warren bypass – use LSV to bypass deep venous blockage – no longer used

NOTES

Post-phlebitic limbs:

- 90% are due to reflux following DVT
- 10% are due to obstruction following DVT

FURTHER READING

Hopkins N F, Wolfe J H (1992) ABC of vascular diseases: deep venous insufficiency. *BMJ* **304**: 107.

CASE 120   GANGRENE   **

INSTRUCTION

'Examine this gentleman's legs.'

APPROACH

Expose the patient and examine the legs (*see* Case 111).

VITAL POINTS

Look

- Note the appearance of gangrene which often begins between the toes
- Comment on whether the gangrene is wet or dry
- Wet gangrene is due to either acute ischaemia or local trauma, and may be complicated by infection
- Wet gangrene usually has an ill-defined, spreading edge
- Skin blistering may occur
- A line of demarcation gradually appears between the viable and dead tissue – if this has occurred, the gangrene is 'dry' and the dead tissue may eventually fall off (autoamputation)
- Continue to comment on the other features of peripheral vascular disease (*see* Case 111)

Feel

Palpate the peripheral pulses and check for temperature differences between the legs (*see* Case 111).

Finish your examination here

QUESTION

(a) What are the causes of gangrene?

Gangrene is the result of irreversible tissue necrosis and has a number of causes:

- Diabetes (the commonest cause)
- Embolus and thrombosis – both leading to acute limb ischaemia, mesenteric infarction, critical limb ischaemia, 'trashing' of feet
- Raynaud's syndrome – *see* Case 121
- Thromboangiitis obliterans (Buerger's disease)– *see* Case 127
- Ergot poisoning
- Vessel injury secondary to extreme cold, heat, trauma or pressure
- Drug-induced, e.g. warfarin

ADVANCED QUESTION

(a) What is Fournier's gangrene?

- Rare necrotizing subcutaneous infection involving the scrotum, penis and perineum
- Scrotum is red and swollen with crepitus on palpation due to dermal gangrene
- Organisms responsible are usually coliforms and anaerobes

** RAYNAUD'S SYNDROME   CASE 121

INSTRUCTION

'Look at this lady's hands and ask her few questions.'

APPROACH

The examiner will often use a leading question like this in order to stimulate a spot diagnosis and lead to some supplemental questions. In this situation, the key is to ascertain the presence of the central clinical features (in this case of Raynaud's) and then to try to identify any precipitating features.

VITAL POINTS

Ask questions at the same time as looking at the hands:

- What is the main problem you have with your hands?
- When does this symptom occur?
- Is it precipitated by any specific weather conditions?
- Can you describe the colour changes your fingers go through during these episodes?

Look

- Note that the pathology is usually bilateral
- In between acute attacks, the skin may be dry and red, especially around the tips of the fingers, and the nails brittle
- Also note any ulcers or gangrene on the pulps

Feel

- The radial pulse is normal

> TOP TIP
> The mnemonic **WBC** may help you recall the order of the skin colour changes of the fingers seen in Raynaud's:
>
> **W**hite – blanching of digits
> **B**lue – cyanosis and pain
> **C**rimson – reactive hyperaemia – fingers turn red in colour

Finish your examination here

Completion

Tell the examiner you would ask about symptoms and look for signs of the secondary causes of Raynaud's.

QUESTIONS

(a) What is the pathogenesis of Raynaud's syndrome?

- If the vessels are normal in calibre, the clinical features may be caused by relatively overactive alpha receptors in the wall, leading to abnormal smooth muscle contraction or changes in elasticity
- Alternatively, there may be a fixed obstruction in the vessel wall, which reduces the distal flow and thus renders the digits susceptible to the effects of cold

(b) What are the predisposing factors?

The causes can be divided into primary and secondary:

- Primary Raynaud's (also known as Raynaud's disease) is due to vasomotor malformation
- Secondary Raynaud's occurs as a consequence of pathology affecting the vessel wall

In general the secondary causes, especially when related to connective tissue diseases, cause more severe problems with necrosis and gangrene.

The secondary causes can be remembered using the mnemonic **BADCaT**:

Blood disorders, e.g. polycythaemia
Arterial, e.g. atherosclerosis, thromboangiitis obliterans
Drugs, e.g. beta blockers, oral contraceptive pill
Connective tissues disorders, e.g. rheumatoid arthritis, systemic lupus erythematosis, scleroderma, polyarteritis nodosa
Trauma, e.g. vibration injury

ADVANCED QUESTION

What are the treatment options for Raynaud's?

Non-surgical:

- Use of gloves and discontinuing any predisposing drugs, e.g. beta blockers
- Using warm pads in gloves and socks in the winter
- Encourage patients to stop smoking

Medical (used with variable success):

- Calcium channel blockers, e.g. nifedipine
- Prostacyclin analogues
- Alpha blockers
- 5HT antagonists

Surgical:

- Cervical sympathectomy and amputation of the affected phalanges
- Cervical sympathectomy may not be a permanent solution and may only relieve symptoms for 2 years or less
- Amputate only if digits are threatened with gangrene

> *Maurice Raynaud (1834–1881)* was a physician in Paris and he described the differences between primary Raynaud's disease and secondary Raynaud's phenomenon in his MD thesis at the age of 28.

FURTHER READING

Block J A, Sequeira W (2001) Raynaud's phenomenon. *Lancet* **357**(9273): 2042–8.

http://www.nhlbi.nih.gov/health/public/blood/other/raynaud.htm – information for patients

http://members.aol.com/Raynauds/ – homepage of the Raynaud's foundation

CASE 122   NEUROPATHIC ULCER   **

INSTRUCTION

'Examine this lady's feet.'

APPROACH

As previously (see Case 110)

VITAL POINTS

Look

Observe the characteristic features of a neuropathic ulcer:

Site:

- They are usually found over the pressure areas, over the metatarsal heads on the sole of the foot and the balls of the toes; they can also occur on the heel

Shape:

- Irregular, correspond to the shape of the pressure point that has become exposed

Edge and base:

- Clean edge
- Base may be deep, with exposure of bone and tendon

Surrounding skin:

- The surrounding skin has a normal blood supply and therefore looks normal

Feel

- Feel the temperature of the surrounding skin, which is expected to be normal
- The peripheral pulses are usually normal
- Test the sensation over the dermatomes using light touch and pinprick, note the absence of sensation around the ulcer and describe the extent of the sensory abnormality

Finish your examination here

TOP TIP
It can be difficult to distinguish between an ischaemic and neuropathic ulcer, however, neuropathic ulcers are:

- Painless
- Associated with normal appearance of the surrounding skin
- Associated with local sensory loss

Completion

Tell the examiner that you would perform a complete neurological examination, including cranial and peripheral nerves.

QUESTIONS

(a) What are the causes of neuropathic ulcers?

They can be caused by any disease that leads to a peripheral sensory neuropathy, or by causes of spinal cord disease. Causes of peripheral neuropathy include:

- Idiopathic (50–60%)
- Systemic diseases:
  - diabetes
  - vasculitis (SLE)
  - hypothyroidism
  - vitamin B12 deficency
- Drugs and toxins:
  - prescribed drugs (amiodarone)
  - alcohol
  - toxins
- Infections:
  - TB, leprosy
  - HIV
- Carcinomas, especially in lung cancer and polycythaemia rubra vera

(b) Why do these ulcers form?

Peripheral neuropathy leads to a slowly progressive sensory loss, with numbness and tingling of the feet and sometimes also hands. The sensory loss is often glove-and-stocking in distribution and may also be associated with motor impairment. The impact of the sensory loss is that damage over the pressure areas is not noticed by the patient. Progressive skin loss and ulceration may occur.

FURTHER READING

Phillips T J (1999) Successful methods of treating leg ulcers. The tried and true, plus the novel and new. *Postgrad Med* **105**(5): 159–61, 165–6, 173–4.

http://www.skinwound.com/online_training_manual/neuropathic_wounds.htm – guide to neuropathic ulcers

NOTE – Rarer causes of leg ulceration

The following causes of leg ulcers may also be encountered in the clinical examination, a couple of characteristics are listed for each type:

Tuberculosis:

- Undermined edge
- Shallow ulcer

Pyoderma gangrenosum:

- Undermined edge
- Violaceous
- Necrotic ulcer with hypertrophic margins

Syphilis:

- Gumma of tertiary syphilis has a typical punched-out ulcer, over the anterior surface of the lower leg and has a yellow coloured 'wash leather' base
- 'Scalloped' border

Arteriovenous fistulae:

- Ulcer is distal to the fistula
- Shallow indolent ulcers

Rheumatoid arthritis:

- Necrotizing vasculitis
- Purpuric, haemorrhagic bullae

Squamous cell carcinoma:

- Rolled or raised edge
- Often on sun-damaged skin

Sickle cell disease:

- Small, punched-out ulcers
- Often over medial aspect of lower leg

CASE 123   LYMPHOEDEMA   ★ ★

INSTRUCTION

'Examine this lady's legs.'

APPROACH

Expose the patient's legs, preserving her dignity.

VITAL POINTS

Look

- The legs may be grossly swollen, with no particular distribution
- Tends to be bilateral
- Note the loss of contour at the ankle which causes a 'buffalo hump' appearance on the dorsum of the foot

- There may be lichenified fronds on the toes and the skin looks thick and indurated (hyperkeratosis, lichenification and peau d'orange)
- Yellow discolouration of nails

Palpate

- Determine whether or not the oedema is pitting in nature
- Initially the oedema is characteristically pitting but later it stops pitting as tissue resistance increases
- Palpate the groin for inguinal lymphadopathy (which may be present)

Finish your examination here

> TOP TIP
> The commonest cause of unilateral ankle oedema is venous disease; lymphoedema is much more commonly bilateral.

Completion

Tell the examiner you would:

- Examine the jugular venous pulse, heart and lungs to exclude right-sided cardiac failure
- Palpate the liver to identify hepatomegaly
- Ask the patient some questions to determine any hereditary conditions that predispose to lymphoedema

QUESTION

(a) What is the differential diagnosis of swollen legs?

Lymphoedema can be similar in appearance to any other cause of swollen legs, but tends to be bilateral:

- Central causes include right heart failure, hypoalbuminaemia, nephrotic syndrome and hypothyroidism
- Peripheral (local) causes are usually venous disease such as deep vein thrombosis, Klippel–Trenaunay syndrome, chronic venous insufficiency or post-phlebitic limb (*see* Case 109, 110 and 119)
- Rare causes are angio-oedema, arteriovenous malformations (Parkes–Weber syndrome, multiple AV fistulae) and hemi-hypertrophy

ADVANCED QUESTIONS

(b) What is the difference between primary and secondary lymphoedema?

Primary lymphoedema refers to congenital disease or primary lymphatic failure. It is three times more common in women and the pathology originates from within the lymphatics. It is also known as Milroy's disease.

Secondary lymphoedema can be classified according to the cause:

- Malignancy – infiltration of nodes; may also cause a chylothorax or chylous ascites when this occurs in nodes in the thorax and abdomen.
- Infections, e.g. filiaris (infection by the *Wuchereria Bancrofti* worm), tuberculosis
- Post surgery or radiotherapy such as axillary dissection in breast surgery and inguinal irradiation

(b) What are the treatment options?

Non-surgical:

- Grade III compression stockings to apply 40 mmHg pressure at the ankles
- Intermittent pneumatic compression device
- Cellulitis should be treated
- Advise patient to elevate their leg as much as possible and stress the importance of cleanliness and careful chiropody

Limb elevation reduces intravascular hydrostatic pressure and the stockings increase extracellular hydrostatic pressure, together reducing the level of tissue oedema. These measures can be very successful but patient motivation is key and it may take some time for the results to become apparent.

Surgical:

- Used rarely – the results tend overall to be poor
- More likely to be successful where there is discrete occlusion of the lymphatics
- Options include:
  - direct lymphovenous anastamosis
  - stripping a piece of small intestine mucosa, exposing the rich submucosal plexus – this can then be used to replace a leg lymph node which then forms new connections with distal lymphatics in order to drain the leg
  - debulking to reduce the volume of the leg – Homans' procedure is an example of such an operation. Flaps are raised above and below the knee (beginning on the medial side and then returning to surgery later if required to complete the lateral flap) and strips of subcutaneous tissue are removed before the flap is sutured. If the skin is in poor condition, a different operation, which excises the skin in addition to the soft tissues, can be performed and the skin covered with a split skin graft (Charles' procedure).

Joseph Bancroft (1836–1894). Surgeon to the General Hospital, Brisbane, Australia.

John Homans (1877–1954). Professor of Clinical Surgery, Harvard Medical School, Boston. He also described Homans' sign, which occurs when passive dorsiflexion of the foot gives pain in the calf in the presence of a deep vein thrombosis.

WF Milroy (1855–1942). North American physician.

FURTHER READING

Cohen S R, Payne D K, Tunkel R S (2001) Lymphedema: strategies for management. *Cancer* **92**(4 Suppl): 980–7.

Rockson S G (2001) Lymphedema. *Am J Med* **110**(4): 288–95.

http://www.lymphoedema.org/lsn/ – information and support network for patients.

http://www.cancerbacup.org.uk/info/lymphoedema.htm – online booklet from CancerBACUP about lymphoedema.

** HYPERHIDROSIS CASE 124

INSTRUCTION

'Examine this patient's hands.'

APPROACH

Expose to the elbows and ask the patient to place his hands palm upwards on a pillow (if available).

VITAL POINTS

Describe the presence of excessive sweat on the palmar surface of both hands, confirming this by palpation.

Finish your examination here

Completion

Say that you would like to:

- Examine the axillae, groins and soles of the feet for excessive sweating
- Enquire about the social effects of the symptoms
- Exclude underlying causes (see below)

QUESTIONS

(a) What is the differential diagnosis?

- Anxiety
- Hyperthyroidism
- Hyperhidrosis erythematosus traumatica – rare occupational form where a vibratory surface, (e.g. capstan lathe) produces excessive sweating of the skin on contact
- Phaeochromocytoma

(b) How do you treat this condition?

- Reassurance – if symptoms are not distressing to the patient
- Medical – aluminium hexachloride solution painting for axillary hyperhidrosis
- Surgical:
  - axillary – excise hair-bearing skin/intradermal Botulinum A neurotoxin (Botox) – this has a 62% cure rate
  - palmar – cervical sympathectomy (T2–T4) via thoracoscopic approach – this has a 98% cure rate
  - plantar – lumbar sympathectomy

(c) What side-effects would you warn this patient about if considering cervical sympathectomy?

- Excessive dryness of skin
- Compensatory sweating around trunk (in up to 50% of patients)
- Horner's syndrome (a consequence of damage to the stellate ganglion) – 0.1%
- Pneumothorax/haemothorax
- Important to warn of the risks of a general anaesthetic for what may be largely a cosmetic problem

ADVANCED QUESTIONS

(a) What other part of the body can be affected by hyperhidrosis?

The face can be affected in patients with:

- Syringomyelia
- Frey's syndrome (*see* Case 21)

FURTHER READING

Chiou T S, Chen S C (1999) Intermediate-term results of endoscopic transaxillary T2 sympathectomy for primary palmar hyperhidrosis. *Br J Surg* **86**(1): 45–7.

Glogau R G (1998) Botulinum A neurotoxin for axillary hyperhidrosis. No sweat Botox. *Dermatol Surg* **24**(8): 817–9.

http://www.parsec.it/summit/hyper1e.htm – a general guide to hyperhidrosis.
http://personal.msy.bellsouth.net/msy/k/a/kaikai/ – hyperhidrosis sufferers home page (what to tell your patients).

INSTRUCTION

'Examine this gentleman's abdomen.'

APPROACH

Expose the patient's abdomen and begin your examination as per Case 43. The examiner will probably move you on to inspection.

VITAL POINTS

Inspection

Note the presence of surgical scars over the abdomen and accurately describe their position.

Palpate

- When palpating the abdomen think carefully about whether there is an incisional hernia over the scars
- Describe the pulsatile swelling underneath one of the scars
- Define the anatomical position of the swelling – midline/lateral etc and ascertain the artery it is most likely to be associated with (aorta/common iliac/external iliac)
- Continue on to palpate the femoral pulses

Auscultate

There may be a bruit over the swelling.

Finish your examination here

QUESTIONS

(a) What is the difference between a false and a true aneurysm?

- An aneurysm (*see* Case 115) is a localized dilatation of a blood vessel (Fig. 42)
- A true aneurysm involves all layers of the arterial wall
- A false aneurysm follows a partial laceration of the vessel wall, causing blood to leak out of the vessel into the surrounding tissues
- A false aneurysm is the same as a pulsating haematoma and is most common in the femoral artery
- Fibrous tissue forms around the haematoma and then contracts, producing a false sac which contains thrombus but remains connected to the lumen of the damaged vessel

- Pulsation transmitted from the artery tends to increase the size of the cavity with time

(b) What are the causes of a false aneurysm?

- Traumatic
- Iatrogenic
  - following angiography, blood continues to leak from the puncture site (easy to repair with suture to arterial wall)
  - following bypass, e.g. femoropopliteal, is often associated with infection (more complex and often need vein patch to reconstruct)

(c) What are the treatment options?

- Ultrasound compression of the false aneurysm
- Thrombin injection
- Surgical repair
- Observation and review

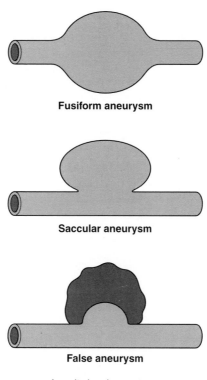

Fusiform aneurysm

Saccular aneurysm

False aneurysm

A cavity in a haematoma
which connects with the
lumen of the artery

Fig. 42   The types of aneurysm.

* THORACIC OUTLET OBSTRUCTION   CASE 126

INSTRUCTION

'Examine this lady's right arm.'

APPROACH

Expose the patient's arm and shoulder, also taking care to expose the contralateral arm.

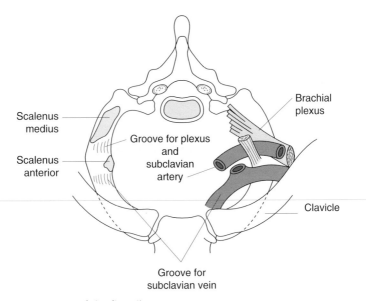

Fig. 43   Anatomy of the first rib.

VITAL POINTS

Look

- Inspect the arm from the anterior and posterior
- Note the presence of oedema, cyanosis or pallor due to REDUCED VENOUS OUTFLOW from the arm – the patient may describe the appearance or worsening of these symptoms on exercise
- Inspect the hand especially carefully, with the hand resting on a white pillow noting the possible ARTERIAL COMPLICATIONS of thoracic outlet syndrome:
  – patchy gangrene of the tips of the fingers and palm
  – fingertip necrosis
- Continue by examining for wasting of the small muscles of the hand (T1 distribution), a feature caused by the NEUROLOGICAL DEFICIT from the obstruction

Palpation

- Palpate the neck, in thin people – there may be a bony swelling of the cervical rib above the clavicle in the supraclavicular fossa
- A pulsatile mass might be present (due to post-stenotic dilatation)
- If there is any evidence of oedema, palpate this and note that it is characteristically pitting in nature
- The radial pulse is usually present and normal

Ausculation

- There might be a bruit over the subclavian artery (Fig. 43)

Sensation

- Test sensation in the dermatomes of the arm specifically – there may be sensory loss over the T1 region, along the medial aspect of the arm around the elbow joint

Finish your examination here

QUESTIONS

(a) What is the differential diagnosis of thoracic outlet obstruction?

This is often a difficult diagnosis to make because the clinical signs are the result of a mix of arterial, venous and neurological complications of the obstruction.

Arterial symptoms (fingertip gangrene, necrosis) are more commonly due to:

- Raynaud's syndrome (*see* Case 121)
- Thromboangiitis obliterans (*see* Case 127)
- Takayasu's arteritis

Venous symptoms (oedema, cyanosis or pallor of the arm) may be caused by:

- Axillary vein thrombosis
- Damage to axillary drainage following surgery (such as axillary dissection in breast surgery)

Neurological symptoms may be due to:

- Cervical spondylosis
- Pancoast's tumour
- Cervical disc protrusions
- Ulnar nerve neuropathy

(b) What investigations may help to confirm the diagnosis?

- There may be a cervical rib or prominent transverse process on the chest X-Ray or thoracic outlet views
- Doppler examination may be useful in quantifying the postural changes and post-stenotic dilatation

- Arteriograms of the subclavian artery may show a marked kink in the artery or even the vein, and sometimes there is a localised aneurysm at the site of the narrowing

(c) What is the pathogenesis of thoracic outlet obstruction?

Congenital:

- Usually due to a cervical rib (arising from the seventh cervical vertebra) and the subclavian artery is compressed between the rib and either the scalenus anterior muscle or the clavicle

Acquired:

- The obstruction may also follow a fractured clavicle, hypertrophy of the scalene muscles, or occasionally a pathological enlargement of the first rib

> *Mikito Takayasu (1860–1938)* was a Japanese surgeon, describing an obliterative arteritis affecting the subclavian and carotid arteries of young Asian women.
> *Henry Khunrath Pancoast (1875–1939).* Professor of Roentgenology, University of Pennsylvania, Philadelphia, USA.

FURTHER READING

Parziale J R, Akelman E, Weiss A P, Green A (2000) Thoracic outlet syndrome. *Am J Orthop* **29**(5): 353–60.

---

* THROMBOANGIITIS OBLITERANS (BUERGER'S DISEASE)   CASE 127

INSTRUCTION

'Look at this man's legs and ask him some questions.'

APPROACH

Expose the patient and examine the legs as for any vascular case (*see* Case 111).

VITAL POINTS

Look

- Nicotine staining of the fingers.
- The patient may complain of chronic paronychia and early ulcers that heal poorly
- There may be a history of intermittent claudication

- Note the presence of distal gangrene and other appearances of chronic ischaemia in the feet, and of erythema nodosum
- Patients often have multiple amputations

Feel

When examining the pulses, the typical pattern is that the femoral and popliteal pulses are present and the foot pulses are absent.

Finish your examination here

QUESTIONS

(a) What is the pathogenesis of thromboangiitis obliterans?

- It is a collagen vascular disease, caused by infiltrate of plasma cells into the arterial wall
- This leads to luminal thrombosis and affects small and medium-sized arteries of the lower limb
- Eventually, collagen is deposited and forms a thick fibrous coat
- Heavy smoking is very strongly associated with this condition

(b) What specific investigations would you perform?

- Collagen antibodies are present in 45% of patients
- There is an association with HLA-B5
- Angiography has typical appearances of normal proximal vessels with distal occlusion and 'corkscrew' collaterals

---

Leo Buerger (1879–1943). North American urologist

FURTHER READING

Olin J W (2000) Thromboangiitis obliterans (Buerger's disease). *N Engl J Med* **343**(12): 864–9.

INSTRUCTION

'Look at this lady's neck and tell me what the problem is.'

VITAL POINTS

Look

- Note the tortuous, visible, dilated veins overlying the chest wall and neck – these veins would not be expected to be compressible
- The face may be plethoric and swollen
- Comment if the patient is dyspnoeic at rest

Finish your examination here

Completion

Tell the examiner you would examine the patient further to find a cause for the obstruction, including looking for peripheral stigmata of lung carcinoma (e.g. nicotine stains, digital clubbing and Horner's syndrome), lymphadenopathy and examining the chest.

QUESTIONS

(a) What are the causes of superior vena cava (SVC) obstruction?

Causes can be divided into pathology within and outside the SVC. Within the SVC obstruction tends to be as a consequence of thrombosis within intravenous jugular or subclavian lines (CVP lines), especially when hyperosmolar solutions are infused for feeding.

Outside the superior vena cava (compression from pathologies in adjacent structures):

- Carcinoma of the lung
- Lymphoma
- Carcinoma of the thyroid
- Aortic aneurysm
- Mediastinal goitre
- Mediastinal fibrosis
- Constrictive pericarditis

(b) How can the extent of the obstruction be determined?

- An intravenous injection of contrast into the veins in the arm can illustrate the degree of obstruction
- A CT scan of the thorax may demonstrate the cause of the obstruction and the length of SVC affected

ADVANCED QUESTIONS

(a) How can thrombosis secondary to a jugular feeding line be treated?

In this situation the patient can be treated with thrombolysis, angioplasty and stenting of the SVC.

Johann Friedrich Horner (1831–1886). Professor of Ophthalmology in Zurich who described Horner's syndrome – ipsilateral ptosis, miosis, hypohidrosis and enophthalmos due to damage to the cervical sympathetic chain.

William Harvey (1578–1657). Physician at St Bartholomew's Hospital, London and President of the Royal College of Physicians. He gave the first account of the circulation of blood in his book *De Motu Cordis* in 1628, although he first spoke of its existence in 1616.

FURTHER READING

Markman M (1999) Diagnosis and management of superior vena cava syndrome. *Cleve Clin J Med* **66**(1): 59–61.

NOTES

There are two other conditions where dilated veins can be observed across the trunk:

- Inferior vena cava obstruction, where the dilated veins occur across the lower abdomen; the commonest cause is intra-abdominal malignancy
- Caput medusa, dilated veins around a portosystemic anastamosis in the umbilical veins.

The three causes of dilated abdominal wall veins can be distinguished by the direction of flow within the dilated veins. This is detected by placing two fingers on the vein, sliding one finger along the vein to empty it and then releasing one finger, watching to see which direction the empty segment fills (Harvey's test).

In relation to the umbilicus:

- In SVC obstruction the direction of flow above the umbilicus is downwards
- In IVC obstruction the direction of flow below the umbilicus is upwards
- In caput medusa the direction of flow is away from the umbilicus (both below and above)

* CAROTID ARTERY ANEURYSM AND DILATED COMMON CAROTID ARTERY

CASE 129

INSTRUCTION

'Examine this patient's neck.'

APPROACH

Expose the patient and proceed as for the neck exam (*see* Case 6).

VITAL POINTS

Inspect

- A pulsatile swelling can be noted in the line of the carotid artery at the base of the neck
- It is normally unilateral

Palpate

- The aneurysm is firm and expansile

Auscultate

- A bruit may be heard

Finish your examination here

Completion

Say that you would:

- Look for neurological associations (ipsilateral Horner's syndrome and focal neurological signs caused by embolization of the aneurysm)
- Examine for other cardiovascular associations (measuring the blood pressure, examining the peripheral pulses and heart)

QUESTIONS

(a) How would the patient be investigated?

Other risk factors and cardiovascular disease elsewhere would be excluded and the neck imaged with a duplex scan or occasionally an intravenous digital subtraction angiogram.

(b) What is the cause of these aneurysms?

- True aneurysms are uncommon and are generally caused by atherosclerosis, and occasionally by dissection, trauma, previous carotid surgery or infection

- When a true aneurysm has been excluded, the patient can be reassured and discharged
- Dilated, tortuous common carotid arteries are much more common – the artery is kinked or coiled and there is a prominent carotid bifurcation

CASE 130   LYMPHANGIOMA *

INSTRUCTION

'Examine this gentleman's neck.'

APPROACH

Begin to examine the neck as described in Case 6. These are usually found in childhood and rarely present in younger adults; they are extremely rare in older adults.

VITAL POINTS

Look

- There is a swelling above the clavicle in the posterior triangle of the neck

Feel

- The swelling feels soft and smooth
- More solid areas may be palpable within the mass
- Characteristically brilliantly transilluminable (because it is full of lymph)
- The skin overlying the lump is normal

Finish your examination here

QUESTIONS

(a) What is the origin of lymphangiomas?

Fifty percent are present at birth and they are thought to represent a congenital abnormality during the evolution of embryonic lymph nodes into the adult type.

(b) How are they classified?

Lymphangiomas can be:

- Cystic (cystic hygroma, as in this case – for further information, *see* Case 37)
- Solid or diffuse – may involve any part of the body, usually present at birth; local overgrowth of tissues and bone may occur which can render surgical correction extremely difficult

- Cutaneous (lymphangioma circumscriptum) present as groups of multiple small transparent blisters lying close to each other. They are usually not present at birth but develop later. They tend to be cosmetically more disfiguring and also ooze fluid or bleed frequently; early surgical treatment is therefore warranted. An ellipse of skin and underlying subcutaneous tissue should be excised.

FURTHER READING

Orvidas L J, Kasperbauer J L (2000) Pediatric lymphangiomas of the head and neck. *Ann Otol Rhinol Laryngol* **109**(4): 411–21.

---

* ARTERIOVENOUS FISTULA   CASE 131

INSTRUCTION

'Examine this gentleman's right wrist and tell me the diagnosis.'

APPROACH

- Expose the patient's hands and place them palm upward on a white pillow if available
- Check that both hands and forearms are exposed to compare one side with the other

VITAL POINTS

Inspect

- There is a swelling over the distal forearm, just proximal to the wrist joint
- Describe this swelling as for any other lump (*see* Case 1)
- The arteriovenous (AV) fistula may have been surgically created, i.e. a Cimino–Bresica fistula for haemodialysis in patients with chronic renal failure (in which case there should be a precise scar over the skin) or it could be traumatic, or occasionally congenital
- The lump may be pulsatile

Palpate

- Check that the patient does not have any pain and then palpate the mass
- There is also a thrill palpable

Auscultate

- The lump has a machinery murmur in systole

Finish your examination here

Completion

Tell the examiner you would examine the rest of the patient to try to determine why the fistula had been formed in the first place.

ADVANCED QUESTIONS

(a) How is a Cimino-Bresica arteriovenous fistula fashioned?

- The procedure can be performed under a regional (brachial plexus) or local block
- A longitudinal incision 3–4 cm in length is made over the distal third of the forearm midway between the radial artery and the cephalic vein
- The cephalic vein is mobilized and tributaries divided
- The radial artery is also identified and dissected and a longitudinal venotomy and parallel longitudinal arteriotomy performed
- Fine non-absorbable sutures are used to join the two
- The distal cephalic vein is ligated altogether

(b) What are the specific complications of a Cimino–Bresica fistula?

- Thrombosis during or just after haemodialysis, which may be due to relative hypotension and damage to the intima of the vein
- Venous hypertension in the hand causes swelling and ischaemia of the fingertips. This should be avoided by the ligation of the distal vein segment
- High-output cardiac failure secondary to massive run-off through the fistula
- Pseudoaneurysm formation

(c) How would you determine clinically the degree of shunt caused by a large fistula?

- The Branham–Nicoladoni sign indicates the degree of shunting and cardiac impairment resulting from a large AV fistula
- The carotid pulse is palpated and then a tourniquet placed around the proximal affected limb and inflated above systolic pressure
- The pulse during the period when the tourniquet is inflated is compared with the pulse beforehand
- Normally an AV fistula causes a hyperdynamic circulation – sinus tachycardia may be present
- When the fistula is cut off from the circulation, this is corrected and so the pulse will slow during the test
- This indicates the presence of a left-to-right shunt

M. J. Bresica. Contemporary renal physician, VA Hospital, New York.
J. E. Cimino. Contemporary renal physician, VA Hospital, New York.
H. H. Branham. 19th Century North American surgeon.

Other types of arteriovenous fistula – these are all rare

(a) Congenital:

- Most commonly occur in the head, neck and limbs
- They can lead to AV aneurysms
- In the head, they most commonly involve the superficial temporal artery
- If the overlying mucous membrane or skin ulcerates, the fistula may haemorrhage
- Small asymptomatic fistulae may be treated expectantly or occasionally with therapeutic embolization
- Surgical options include occlusion of the feeding vessel and excision of the fistula and surrounding aneurysm if present, or radiological embolization

(b) Multiple arteriovenous fistulae (Parkes–Weber syndrome)

- These are almost always in the limbs and present with an overall increase in the size of the affected limb
- The limb has the appearances of extensive varicose veins
- These are very often complicated by severe lipodermatosclerosis and ulceration
- Bruits and thrills may be present
- The Branham–Nicoladoni sign is normally positive (see above)
- Usually it is impossible to excise or embolize each individual fistula unless they are all derived from a single peripheral artery

(c) Traumatic:

- May follow a simultaneous partial laceration through a vein and artery lying in apposition
- Occur several days after the injury
- More common after open injuries
- The patient may notice a thrill or buzzing
- The other situation where this may occur is following cannulation of vessels by radiologists or cardiologists
- These fistulae normally need to be explored, the vessels separated and the defect closed

FURTHER READING

http://www.niddk.nih.gov/health/kidney/pubs/kidney-failure/vascular-access/vascular-access.htm – information on vascular access for haemodialysis, with diagrams

CASE 132   COARCTATION OF THE AORTA   *

INSTRUCTION

'Examine this gentleman's back and describe the abnormalities you see.'

APPROACH

Expose the patient to the waist, and ask him to stand or sit forward on the side of the bed so that you can examine the back adequately (*see* Case 99)

VITAL POINTS

Look

- Note the large, prominent, tortuous blood vessels running over the left scapula
- Palpate the vessels to demonstrate that they are arteries
- Listen to the vessels and confirm the presence of a systolic murmur

Finish your examination here

Completion

- Tell the examiner you would compare the pulses in the arms and legs – the upper limb pulses are much stronger than the leg pulses
- The patient is usually hypertensive
- You would examine for radio-femoral delay and examine the precordium for an ejection systolic murmur heard over the left sternal edge

QUESTIONS

(a) What is the pathophysiology of coarctation?

- The aorta is narrowed below the origin of the left subclavian artery and therefore blood flow to the abdomen and legs is reduced
- The prominent vessels over the back are large collaterals that have developed to bypass the obstruction and supply the legs
- The collaterals form between branches of the subclavian artery, especially the internal mammary and scapular vessels, which feed the intercostals from the third rib down

(b) What investigations would be helpful in confirming the diagnosis?

- Notching on the underside of the ribs may be seen on a chest X-ray (CXR) – this sign is caused by erosion by the intercostal collateral vessels
- On the CXR the aorta may be abnormal – it contains two bulges – the 'three sign'

- A barium swallow shows the opposite – the 'reverse three sign' in the oesophagus
- An echocardiogram shows the site of the coarctation and may demonstrate concurrent aortic stenosis

ADVANCED QUESTIONS

(a) What associations of coarctation are you aware of?

Coarctation may be associated with:

- Bicuspid aortic valves
- Aortic stenosis
- Aneurysms in the circle of Willis

(b) What are the treatment options?

Non-surgical:

- Investigation and treatment of concurrent abnormalities (present in 50%)
- Management of hypertension

Surgical:

- End-to-end anastomosis, patching and the use of the left subclavian artery as a flap are all surgical options

FURTHER READING

McCrindle B W (1999) Coarctation of the aorta. *Curr Opin Cardiol* **14**(5): 448–52.

---

* ATRIAL FIBRILLATION   CASE 133

INSTRUCTION

'Take this lady's pulse and comment on it.'

VITAL POINTS

- Ask for permission, and then take the patient's right radial pulse and then a central (carotid) pulse
- Rate and rhythm (Table 32) should be ascertained from the radial pulse
- Character and volume are determined from the carotid pulse
- It is often easier to use the thumb to palpate the carotid pulse, but be careful to avoid giving the sensation of strangling the patient by using the right thumb to take the pulse in the left side of the neck

Finish your examination here

Table 32   Assessment of rate, rhythm, character and volume of pulse

Rate	Espressed in beats/minute Count for 15 seconds and multiply beats by 4

Rhythm	Regular or irregular
	If irregular can be regularly or irregularly irregular
	• Regularly irregular:
	  – extrasystoles
	  – sinus arrhythmias (faster in inspiration)
	  – pulsus paradoxus (weaker in inspiration)
	  – pulses alternans (alternating weak and strong beats)
	• Irregularly irregular:
	  – atrial fibrillation (AF)

Character	Rate of increase and decrease of the pressure within the wave of the pulse • Collapsing pulse ('waterhammer pulse') – steep rise then rapid fall is characteristic of aortic regurgitation • Anacrotic pulse – a slow rise and a slow fall in aortic stenosis, as the normal dicrotic notch is lost
Volume	The expansion of the artery with each beat is palpated in the carotid artery • High cardiac output leads to a strong pulse • A patient with severe blood loss and shock has a thready pulse

Completion

Tell the examiner that you would continue to examine the rest of the cardiovascular system and look especially for complications of atrial fibrillation (see below).

QUESTIONS

(a) What are the causes of atrial fibrillation?

Cardiac disease:

- Hypertension
- Myocardial infarction, ischaemia
- Mitral valve disease
- Cardiomyopathy
- Endocarditis

Respiratory disease:

- Pneumonia
- Lung cancer
- Sarcoidosis

Other:
- Hyperthyroidism
- Lone AF where it is not due to any of the causes listed above

(b) What are the complications of atrial fibrillation?

- The major risk is of embolic stroke (4% per year), which results from thrombus accumulating in an inefficiently contracting left atrium
- Emboli can also lodge in the mesenteric vessels, causing intestinal ischaemia
- Patients are also at risk from acute limb ischaemia if emboli lodge in the arteries of the leg

(c) What are the surgical problems associated with atrial fibrillation?

- Anaesthesia is more complicated because of the increased risk of stroke
- In addition, patients with AF may be anticoagulated and if on warfarin, this medication needs to be discontinued prior to elective surgery
- Patients with controlled AF may decompensate following the stress of surgery and in the most severe cases, this can lead to hypotension
- Finally, the underlying cause for the AF, such as ischaemic heart disease, is still present and may contribute further to anaesthetic risk

FURTHER READING

Falk R H (2001) Atrial fibrillation. *N Engl J Med* **344**(14): 1067–78.

INDEX